Inclusive and Barrier-Free Designs for Rehabilitation Engineering

Toshiaki Tanaka
Editor

Inclusive and Barrier-Free Designs for Rehabilitation Engineering

Springer

Editor
Toshiaki Tanaka
Research Center for Advanced Science
and Technology (RCAST) / Institute
of Gerontology (IOG)
The University of Tokyo
Tokyo, Japan

ISBN 978-981-95-5782-0 ISBN 978-981-95-5783-7 (eBook)
https://doi.org/10.1007/978-981-95-5783-7

This Springer imprint is published by the registered company Springer Nature Singapore Pte Ltd.
The registered company address is: 152 Beach Road, #21-01/04 Gateway East, Singapore 189721, Singapore

Foreword

Tohru Ifukube

The growing complexity of health, welfare, and social systems in aging societies has brought renewed attention to the fundamental importance of inclusive and barrier-free design in rehabilitation engineering. As populations diversify in functional needs and social participation becomes increasingly recognized as a core dimension of well-being, the demand for evidence-based, user-centered technological solutions continues to expand. This volume, *Inclusive and Barrier-Free Designs for Rehabilitation Engineering*, offers a timely and academically rigorous contribution to this evolving field.

The chapters collected here span conceptual foundations, methodological developments, and empirical case studies across a wide spectrum of disabilities and functional domains. Early chapters articulate the theoretical basis of inclusive and barrier-free design within clinical and community contexts, while subsequent sections present applied research on visual and motor impairments, mobility support, communication assistance, telerehabilitation, and emerging areas such as para-eSports and virtual reality–based training. This comprehensive scope reflects the inherently interdisciplinary nature of rehabilitation engineering, integrating perspectives from clinical sciences, assistive technology, ergonomics, design studies, and human–computer interaction.

A notable strength of this volume is its consistent engagement with real-world environments and user experiences. The contributions emphasize that effective assistive technologies must be grounded not only in engineering performance but also in the lived realities, preferences, and aspirations of older adults and persons with disabilities. This aligns with ongoing discussions on accessibility and universal design in Europe and the United States, emphasizing the importance of situating assistive technology development within the broader context of social inclusion.

For researchers, clinicians, and designers, this volume offers both theoretical clarity and practical insight. For policymakers and practitioners, it provides perspectives that may support evidence-informed decision-making in health and social care systems. For students, it serves as an accessible yet academically robust entry point into the growing field of inclusive rehabilitation engineering.

It is anticipated that this book will stimulate further interdisciplinary dialogue, encourage the co-creation of inclusive technological solutions, and contribute to advancing equitable and sustainable rehabilitation practices across diverse societies.

Preface

In recent years, the rapid progression of population aging and the growing recognition of the importance of social participation for people with disabilities have drawn increasing attention to the roles of barrier-free and inclusive design in rehabilitation science and welfare. These concepts extend beyond the mere removal of physical obstacles. They represent essential perspectives for developing products and environments that respond to diverse user needs and circumstances, ensuring that everyone can use them safely and comfortably.

This book, *Inclusive and Barrier-Free Designs for Rehabilitation Engineering*, introduces case studies of assistive device development as well as the design thinking that supports them. Chapter 1 outlines the basic concepts of inclusive and barrier-free design in the medical field and discusses their potential applications in rehabilitation. Chapter 2 explains idea generation methods and development processes for assistive devices based on these approaches. Chapters 3, 4, 5, 6, 7, 8, and 9 present specific case studies addressing visual and motor impairments, mobility support, and assistance for individuals with hearing or speech disorders, including both technical details and usability evaluations. These chapters provide practical insights that go beyond theoretical discussion.

A distinctive feature of this book is its focus not only on the technologies themselves but also on the processes behind them—particularly "idea creation" and "user-centered design." For students and early-career researchers, this volume offers valuable guidance on how to conceptualize technologies from inclusive and barrier-free perspectives. At the same time, the book is intended to be accessible to families caring for older adults or persons with disabilities, to professionals in medical, welfare, and caregiving services, and to all others who support social participation.

The most important perspective emphasized throughout is that technological development must always be grounded in the activities of daily living (ADL) and the quality of life (QOL) desired by elderly or disabled individuals. To achieve this, it is vital to observe real-life environments, to experience daily situations firsthand, and to listen carefully to the voices of those directly involved. Such engagement forms the foundation for envisioning and creating truly necessary assistive technologies.

Finally, I would like to express my heartfelt gratitude to all who contributed to this book. In particular, I owe special thanks to Professor Tohru Ifukube, a leading authority in welfare engineering, for his long-standing guidance; to Professor Marilyn Moffat of New York University, whose instruction in research methodology in physical therapy provided a strong foundation; and to Professor Masaaki Takahashi, who conveyed with passion the significance and excellence of kinesiology research in the field of physical therapy.

Tokyo, Japan Toshiaki Tanaka

Contents

Contributors

Naomi Esashi Non-Profit Organization Piskari, Tokyo, Japan

Shujirou Imaeda Urban Development and Planning Department, Nikken Sekkei Research Institute, Tokyo, Japan

Shinichiro Kumagaya Research Center for Advanced Science and Technology, The University of Tokyo, Tokyo, Japan

Yusuke Maeda School of Health Sciences at Odawara, International University of Health and Welfare, Odawara, Kanagawa, Japan

Rika Miura Non-Profit Organization Piskari, Tokyo, Japan

Takahiro Miura Research Institute on Human and Societal Augmentation (RIHSA), National Institute of Advanced Industrial Science and Technology (AIST), Chiba, Japan

Yasuhiro Nakajima Human Technology Research Division, Industrial Research Institute, Industrial Technology and Environment Research Department, Local Independent Administrative Agency, Hokkaido Research Organization, Hokkaido, Japan

Toshio Otsuki Department of Architecture, Graduate School of Engineering, The University of Tokyo, Tokyo, Japan

Satoshi Shirogane Clinical Evaluation Section, Department of Assistive Technology, Research Institute, National Rehabilitation Center for Persons with Disabilities, Tokorozawa, Japan

Toshiaki Tanaka Research Center for Advanced Science and Technology/Institute of Gerontology, The University of Tokyo, Tokyo, Japan

Ken-ichiro Yabu Research Center for Advanced Science and Technology, The University of Tokyo, Tokyo, Japan
Institute of Gerontology, The University of Tokyo, Tokyo, Japan

Chapter 1
Introduction

Shinichiro Kumagaya and Toshiaki Tanaka

Abstract Around 1980 two global currents—the rise of evidence-based medicine and minority activism for diversity and inclusion—catalysed a decisive turn towards the *social model of disability*. This model reframes disability as a mismatch between individual bodies and social environments rather than as an intrinsic defect. Accordingly, medicine must now redesign its physical, institutional, and cultural systems so that people with disabilities and other marginalized identities can participate fully as patients and colleagues. Closing the resulting health-equity gap requires environments that welcome practitioners with disabilities, embrace user-centred design, and recognize medicine's own "positive powerlessness".

Section 1.2 discusses barrier-free and inclusive design for rehabilitating the elderly and disabled. In Japan, where the population is ageing rapidly and policies promoting the social participation of people with disabilities are advancing, barrier-free and inclusive designs should enhance the quality of life (QOL) of the elderly and disabled by improving their activities of daily living (ADLs) in relation to their living environments. These design approaches start with the concept of "disability" as the basis of design and incorporate social, cultural, and contextual aspects of daily life. Future challenges include coordinating with institutional systems, conducting empirical research, and promoting co-creative design with relevant stakeholders.

S. Kumagaya
Research Center for Advanced Science and Technology, The University of Tokyo, Tokyo, Japan
e-mail: kumashin@bfp.rcast.u-tokyo.ac.jp

T. Tanaka (✉)
Research Center for Advanced Science and Technology/Institute of Gerontology, The University of Tokyo, Tokyo, Japan
e-mail: t.tanaka@iog.u-tokyo.ac.jp; tanaka@bfp.rcast.u-tokyo.ac.jp

T. Tanaka (ed.), *Inclusive and Barrier-Free Designs for Rehabilitation Engineering*,
https://doi.org/10.1007/978-981-95-5783-7_1

1.1 Inclusive Design in Medicine

Shinichiro Kumagaya

1.1.1 Positive Powerlessness: Medicine in the Social Model Era

The disability paradigm shift coincided with my own trajectory. Born with cerebral palsy, I rely on 24-hour personal assistance and an electric wheelchair. After medical school I practised paediatrics and now teach and study tōjisha-kenkyū—unique community-based participatory research by people with disabilities in Japan [1].

In the 1970s Japan, diversity was undervalued, and products, services, and even people were expected to converge on a standardized "average". Children with cerebral palsy were urged to approximate typical development. Early intervention therapies were widely promoted, and like many parents, mine dedicated 5–6 h every day to my rehabilitation—a painful experience for a child [2].

By the late 1970s, however, the oil shocks had ushered in fiscal restraint and a new insistence on proof of efficacy. Sackett's group at McMaster University launched the evidence-based medicine (EBM) movement in 1981, teaching clinicians how to appraise the literature [3]. One by one, cherished therapies were shown to be ineffective, leaving families like mine feeling abandoned.

Yet acknowledging medicine's limits can be empowering. At Urakawa Bethel House, pioneers of tōjisha-kenkyū coined the principle of "positive powerlessness": recognizing that neither professionals nor clients possess all the answers and that new understandings must be co-produced [4].

1.1.1.1 From the Medical to the Social Model

Beginning in the 1980s, rehabilitation merged with worldwide disability activism to replace the medical model—which locates disability within the person—with the social model, which locates it between people and biased environments. Buildings, tools, customs, language, and values built for the majority create "disablement" when they clash with minority bodies and minds. International standards now embed this logic: ISO 9241-210 mandates iterative user involvement across the design life cycle [5], and the US Access Board extends it to diagnostic hardware [6]. Inclusive design and human-factors engineering likewise reject the mythical "average user" [7].

Recognizing that "it was society that needed to be fixed" restored my own hope. The slogan "Nothing About Us Without Us" affirmed the sovereignty of disabled people.

1.1.1.2 Continuing Roles for Medicine

The importance of awareness of one's own powerlessness does not mean that medicine and medical treatment need not play a role for people with disability under the paradigm of the social model of disability.

Knowledge of the body. Detailed biomedical knowledge is still vital for adapting environments to bodily characteristics. Overemphasis on prevention and cure, however, can perpetuate ableism. Research must also pursue well-being and full participation.

Restoring function. Remedies for treatable conditions ("diseases") remain appropriate, but they should be balanced with environmental change.

Treating comorbid illness. People with disabilities also experience ordinary disease. Multi-organ dysfunction is common in cerebral palsy, for example [8].

1.1.2 Inclusive Healthcare and Persistent Health Disparities

Hospitals often lack wheelchair scales, height-adjustable exam tables, or accessible mammography units [9]. For autistic adults, clinical environments can be overwhelmingly sensory [10]. Sign language interpreters, Braille, and easy-to-read formats are still rare.

Physicians also underestimate the quality of life of disabled people [11], contributing to discriminatory decisions in transplantation [12] and pandemic triage [13]. Only 41% of US physicians believe they can deliver equal care to disabled and non-disabled patients; barely half strongly agree that their practice can accommodate such patients [11]. The United Nations [14] and WHO [15] both link these barriers to stark health inequities.

1.1.2.1 Systems Engineering for Equity

Accessible diagnostic equipment standards took effect in 2017 [6], yet procurement and enforcement remain patchy. Disability curricula are likewise scarce: only one quarter of US residents report any such training [16], and assessments seldom test skills such as performing a physical exam with a wheelchair user [17]. Health disparities thus emerge as a classic engineering problem—a poor fit between clinical systems and human variability.

1.1.2.2 Trauma: Past and Present

People with disabilities face elevated risks of violence [18] and of being traumatized by medical encounters themselves. Painful procedures, frightening environments, and disrespectful interactions can produce lasting "medical trauma" [19]. Indigenous health scholars describe historical trauma as adversity transmitted across generations [20]. Disabled communities likewise carry collective memories of exclusion; many patients arrive distrustful and apprehensive. Trauma-informed care must therefore infuse every clinical interaction.

1.1.3 Diversity and Inclusion Inside the Profession

Equal status contact is a proven antidote to prejudice. Working with a colleague who has a disability dismantles stereotypes far more powerfully than treating a disabled patient [21, 22].

1.1.3.1 Physician-Patient Concordance

When patients and physicians share salient identities—race, gender, sexual orientation, or disability—trust, satisfaction, and adherence all improve [23]. Peer support workers, whose expertise stems from lived experience, now extend care beyond the traditional scope.

1.1.3.2 Barriers to Entry

Out-of-date technical standards, inadequate accommodations, and misconceptions still obstruct trainees with disabilities. Cultural norms can strip residents of the chance to learn through failure [24]. The result is a vicious circle: stigma blocks equal contact, and the lack of contact sustains stigma.

1.1.3.3 Global and Japanese Initiatives

International guidelines on disability inclusion in medical education and reasonable accommodation for health professionals debuted in 2020. In Japan, the University of Tokyo launched the Center for Diversity in Medical Education and Research in 2021 and the Inclusive Academia Project in 2020 to dismantle structural barriers, develop peer support roles, and study concordance effects.

Diverse teams also produce better science. Clinicians from varied backgrounds address broader social questions [25, 26] and design studies that benefit more patients [27]. User-researcher positions institutionalize this lived experience expertise.

1.1.4 Conclusion

Grounded in the social model of disability, medicine must relinquish its paternalistic stance, accept its “positive powerlessness”, and collaborate on equal terms with minority users and practitioners. Engineering principles of user-centred, inclusive design provide a practical road map: redesign clinical environments, interfaces, and organizational cultures and cultivate a workforce that mirrors the diversity of the communities served. In so doing, healthcare can transform from a site of exclusion into a living laboratory of equity.

1.2 Barrier-Free and Inclusive Design in Rehabilitation

Toshiaki Tanaka

1.2.1 Introduction

Japanese society is aging at an unprecedented rate. By 2025, it is estimated that people aged 65 and over will account for approximately 30% of the population [28]. Additionally, policies promoting the social participation of persons with disabilities are accelerating. Against this social backdrop, creating environments that are accessible to all, particularly in medical and welfare settings, has become an urgent issue. This paper presents examples of barrier-free and inclusive design applications, particularly in rehabilitation settings, and refers to international case studies (Fig. 1.1).

1.2.2 Barrier-Free Applications in Medical Care

1.2.2.1 Physical Environment Improvements

Barrier-free design is a design philosophy that focuses on removing physical and institutional barriers. In medical facilities, this includes ensuring adequate corridor width, eliminating steps, installing non-slip flooring, and adding tactile paving for the visually impaired. In the United States, the Americans with Disabilities Act imposes strict accessibility standards on hospital design [29]. These standards include toilet and examination room dimensions, signage, and voice guidance system standardization. In Japan, the Ministry of Health, Labor and Welfare published the “Guidelines for Elderly and Disabled-Friendly Medical Facility Development”, which promote similar improvements [30].

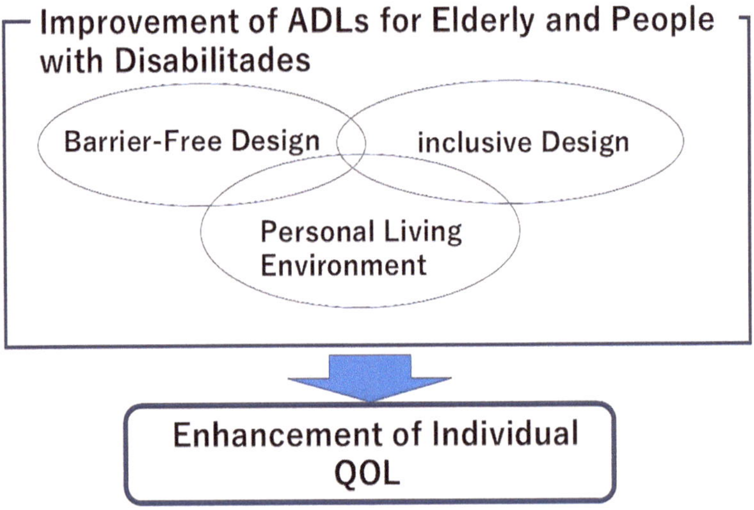

Fig. 1.1 Relationship between barrier-free/inclusive design and ADL/QOL

1.2.2.2 Ensuring Information Accessibility

Effective communication between patients and medical staff is essential in rehabilitation. Therefore, eliminating information barriers is also important. Measures include using simple Japanese, providing explanations with illustrations and videos, and using multilingual electronic devices. For dementia patients and foreign patients, in particular, diversifying communication methods directly improves quality of life (QOL). In the United States, improvements to patient portal site accessibility have been promoted through features such as screen readers and adjustable font sizes [31].

1.2.3 Perspective of Inclusive Design

1.2.3.1 Philosophy and Characteristics

Rather than being designed for specific individuals, inclusive design is "premised on use by diverse people from the start" [28, 32]. In rehabilitation settings, it is necessary to consider patients, caregivers, nurses, physical therapists, family members, and visiting staff as potential users. Unlike universal design, inclusive design uses "disability" as the starting point and incorporates social and cultural backgrounds into the design. As shown in Fig. 1.1, both barrier-free design and inclusive design enhance quality of life (QOL) by improving activities of daily living (ADLs) for the elderly and disabled when integrated into their living environments. In particular, inclusive design starts from the point of "disability" and incorporates social, cultural, and contextual aspects into the design process [33].

1.2.3.2 Specific Examples in Medical Settings

This section presents a case study of the practical application of this design approach in a medical setting, focusing on improvements in hospital navigation and room design for elderly patients with dementia. For these individuals, hospitals are unfamiliar and non-routine spaces that often lead to confusion, making it difficult for them to navigate the wards or recognize their rooms [34].

For instance, in traditional hospital settings, room numbers and wayfinding signs are frequently text based and abstract, making them difficult for patients with cognitive impairments to comprehend. This can hinder their ability to move safely and independently within the facility [35]. In response, one healthcare facility adopted inclusive design measures that incorporated the patients' point of view.

- Color-coded navigation was introduced for each ward to enable intuitive, visually guided wayfinding [36].
- Universal pictograms were used for restrooms, examination rooms, and other facilities to support understanding that does not rely on language or memory function [37].
- Familiar visual elements, such as scenic photos or family pictures preferred by the patient, were displayed on the doors of private rooms to reduce cognitive burden and enhance emotional security [38].
- Furthermore, a workshop-style design process involving patients, their families, nurses, and local welfare personnel was conducted to reflect each individual's lifestyle, habits, and cultural background (e.g. Japanese-style interior design or religious considerations) in the room environment [39].

1.2.4 Integrating Both and the Potential of New Technologies

1.2.4.1 Integrated Perspective of Barrier-Free and Inclusive Design

Barrier-free design aims to "remove obstacles", while inclusive design focuses on "embracing diversity". These two concepts are complementary and should be integrated in stages (Fig. 1.1). The efforts described in Sect. 1.2.3.2 go beyond simply removing physical barriers. They aim to reconstruct living environments that are rooted in "personal identity". This represents a practical example based on the philosophy of inclusive design [33, 39]. As a result, there were fewer incidents of disorientation and anxiety-related behaviours among elderly patients with dementia, and they experienced more stable and peaceful stays in their rooms. This contributes to more consistent activities of daily living (ADL) and a sense of psychological security [34, 40]. Figure 1.1 illustrates how integrating barrier-free and inclusive design into one's living environment enhances both ADL and QOL.

1.2.4.2 Examples of ICT and AI Utilization

In recent years, the introduction of information and communications technology (ICT) and artificial intelligence (AI) technologies has enabled personalized rehabilitation support. Motion analysis systems using AI can visualize rehabilitation effects and provide appropriate feedback. Furthermore, Internet of Things (IoT) monitoring systems and telemedicine technologies allow patients who have difficulty visiting hospitals to receive rehabilitation at home. Incorporating an inclusive user interface (UI)/user experience (UX) design perspective is essential to ensure that these technologies are user-friendly [31, 41].

1.2.5 Future Challenges and Outlook

The following three perspectives will be important in creating future medical environments, along with specific examples:

- Coordination between systems and design
  Building standards, medical fee systems, and designs must be aligned. For example, the Americans with Disabilities Act (ADA) in the United States mandates the accessibility of electronic devices and public facilities [29]. In Japan, the 2021 "Guidelines for Elderly and Disabled-Friendly Medical Facility Development" provide national subsidies for barrier-free improvements [30]. The challenge going forward is how to reflect these efforts in the medical fee system.
- Accumulation of Empirical Research
  A quantitative evaluation of the impact of barrier-free and inclusive design is required. For example, a fall prevention programme for the elderly in the United Kingdom reported a 30% reduction in fall rates after home renovations that incorporated barrier-free design [32]. In Japan, empirical studies have shown improvements in walking speed and reduced psychological burden after steps were removed and tactile paving was installed in welfare facilities [42].
- Promotion of Co-creation Design
  A design process must be established in which designers, medical staff, and stakeholders collaborate. For example, New York City's "Inclusive Design Guidelines" incorporate workshops with disabled stakeholders to reflect user perspectives in public facility design [43]. As community-based integrated care is promoted in Japan, there are increasing examples of involving dementia patients and families in designing cafés and rehabilitation facilities.

1.2.6 Conclusion

Barrier-free and inclusive design philosophies aim to create a "non-exclusive" society, not just "considerations". To improve the quality of life for the elderly and disabled, these ideas must be introduced into rehabilitation settings to create a society where everyone can receive medical care with peace of mind.

References

1. Ayaya, S., Kitanaka, J.: Tōjisha-kenkyū: Japan's radical alternative to psychiatric diagnosis. Aeon, https://aeon.co/essays/japans-radical-alternative-to-psychiatric-diagnosis (2023)
2. Kumagaya, S.: Night of Rehabilitation [Rihabiri no yoru]. Igaku-shoin (2009)
3. Sackett, D.: How to read clinical journals: I. Why to read them and how to start reading them critically. Can. Med. Assoc. J. **1245**, 555–558 (1981)
4. Mukaiyachi, I.: What is tōjisha-kenkyū (2020)
5. ISO: ISO 9241-210: Ergonomics of Human-System Interaction—Human-Centred Design for Interactive Systems. ISO, Geneva (2019)
6. Architectural and Transportation Barriers Compliance Board: Standards for accessible medical diagnostic equipment. Fed. Regist. **82**(5), 2810–2848 (2017)
7. Clarkson, P.J., Coleman, R.: Inclusive Design for Healthcare. Routledge (2018)
8. Allen, J., Zareen, Z., Doyle, S., Whitla, L., Afzal, Z., Stack, M., Franklin, O., Green, A., James, A., Leahy, T.R., Quinn, S., Elnazir, B., Russell, J., Paran, S., Kiely, P., Roche, E.F., McDonnell, C., Baker, L., Hensey, O., Gibson, L., et al.: Multi-organ dysfunction in cerebral palsy. Front. Pediatr. **9**, 668544 (2021)
9. Sonalkar, S., Chavez, V., McClusky, J., Hunter, T.A., Mollen, C.J.: Gynecologic care for women with physical disabilities: a qualitative study of patients and providers. Women's Health Issues. **30**(2), 136–141 (2020)
10. Stein Duker, L.I., Sadie Kim, H.K., Pomponio, A., Mosqueda, L., Pfeiffer, B.: Examining primary care health encounters for adults with autism Spectrum disorder. Am. J. Occup. Ther. **73**(5), 7305185030p1–7305185030p11 (2019)
11. Iezzoni, L.I., Rao, S.R., Ressalam, J., Bolcic-Jankovic, D., Agaronnik, N.D., Donelan, K., Lagu, T., Campbell, E.G.: Physicians' perceptions of people with disability and their health care. Health Affairs (Project Hope). **40**(2), 297–306 (2021)
12. Statter, M.B., Noritz, G., Committee on Bioethics, Council on Children with Disabilities: Children with intellectual and developmental disabilities as organ transplantation recipients. Pediatrics. **145**(5), e20200625 (2020)
13. Scully, J.L.: Disability, disablism, and COVID-19 pandemic triage. J. Bioeth. Inq. **17**(4), 601–605 (2020)
14. United Nations General Assembly: United Nations 2018 flagship report on disability and development: Realization of the Sustainable Development Goals by, for and with persons with disabilities, UN Doc. A/73/220 (2018)
15. World Health Organization: World report on disability. http://www.who.int/disabilities/world_report/2011/en/index.html, https://toukennet.jp/?page_id=56, https://www.un.org/development/desa/disabilities/publication-disability-sdgs.html (2011)
16. Stillman, M.D., Ankam, N., Mallow, M., Capron, M., Williams, S.: A survey of internal and family medicine residents: assessment of disability-specific education and knowledge. Disabil. Health J. **14**(2), 101011 (2021)

17. Sarmiento, C., Miller, S.R., Chang, E., Zazove, P., Kumagai, A.K.: From impairment to empowerment: a longitudinal medical school curriculum on disabilities. Acad. Med. **91**(7), 954–957 (2016)
18. Hughes, K., Bellis, M.A., Jones, L., Wood, S., Bates, G., Eckley, L., McCoy, E., Mikton, C., Shakespeare, T., Officer, A.: Prevalence and risk of violence against adults with disabilities: a systematic review and meta-analysis of observational studies. Lancet (London, England). **379**(9826), 1621–1629 (2012)
19. De Young, A.C., Paterson, R.S., Brown, E.A., Egberts, M.R., Le Brocque, R.M., Kenardy, J.A., Landolt, M.A., Marsac, M.L., Alisic, E., Haag, A.C.: Topical review: medical trauma during early childhood. J. Pediatr. Psychol. **46**(7), 739–746 (2021)
20. Gone, J.P., Hartmann, W.E., Pomerville, A., Wendt, D.C., Klem, S.H., Burrage, R.L.: The impact of historical trauma on health outcomes for indigenous populations in the USA and Canada: a systematic review. Am. Psychol. **74**(1), 20–35 (2019)
21. Shakespeare, T., Iezzoni, L.I., Groce, N.E.: Disability and the training of health professionals. Lancet (London, England). **374**(9704), 1815–1816 (2009)
22. Shakespeare, T., Kleine, I.: Educating health professionals about disability: a review of interventions. Health Soc. Care Educ. **2**(2), 20–37 (2013)
23. Street, R.L., O'Malley, K.J., Cooper, L.A., Haidet, P.: Understanding concordance in patient-physician relationships: personal and ethnic dimensions of shared identity. Ann. Fam. Med. **6**(3), 198–205 (2008)
24. Kumagaya, S., Kita, K., Ayaya, S.: Research on the effects of Tojisha-Kenkyu on the workplace. Econ. Anal. **203**, 28–58 (2021)
25. Eckstrand, K.L., Eliason, J., St Cloud, T., Potter, J.: The priority of intersectionality in academic medicine. Acad. Med. **91**(7), 904–907 (2016)
26. Tsai, J., Ucik, L., Baldwin, N., Hasslinger, C., George, P.: Race matters? Examining and rethinking race portrayal in preclinical medical education. Acad. Med. **91**(7), 916–920 (2016)
27. Meeks, L.M., Neera, R., Jain, N.R.: Accessibility, Inclusion, and Action in Medical Education: Lived Experiences of Learners and Physicians with Disabilities. Association of American Medical Colleges (2018)
28. Cabinet Office: White Paper on People with Disabilities, 2022 edn. https://www8.cao.go.jp/shougai/whitepaper/r04hakusho/zenbun/index-pdf.html (2022)
29. United States Department of Justice: Americans with Disabilities Act of 1990, as amended. https://www.ada.gov (1990)
30. Ministry of Health, Labour and Welfare: Medical reference materials for elderly care facilities, facilities for people with disabilities, etc. https://www.mhlw.go.jp/stf/seisakunitsuite/bunya/0000077386.html (2021)
31. U.S. General Services Administration: Section 508 standards for electronic and information technology. https://www.section508.gov (2020)
32. Clarkson, J., Coleman, R., Keates, S., Lebbon, C. (eds.): Inclusive Design: Design for the Whole Population. Springer (2003)
33. Clarkson, P.J., Coleman, R., Hosking, I., Waller, S.: Inclusive Design Toolkit. University of Cambridge Engineering Design Centre (2007)
34. Mitchell, L., Burton, E.: Designing dementia-friendly neighbourhoods: helping people with dementia to get out and about. J. Integr. Care. **18**(6), 11–18 (2010). https://doi.org/10.5042/jic.2010.0647
35. Brorsson, A., Ohman, A., Lundberg, S., Nygard, L.: Accessibility in public space as perceived by people with Alzheimer's disease. Dementia. **10**(4), 587–602 (2011)
36. Story, M.F., Mueller, J.L., Mace, R.L.: The Universal Design File: Designing for People of All Ages and Abilities. NC State University, Center for Universal Design (1998)
37. Iwarsson, S., Ståhl, A.: Accessibility, usability and universal design—positioning and definition of concepts describing person–environment relationships. Disabil. Rehabil. **25**(2), 57–66 (2003)

38. Day, K., Carreon, D., Stump, C.: The therapeutic design of environments for people with dementia: a review of the empirical research. The Gerontologist. **40**(4), 397–416 (2000)
39. Lindsay, S., Brittain, K., Jackson, D., Ladha, C., Ladha, K., Olivier, P.: Empathy, participatory design and people with dementia. In: Proceedings of the SIGCHI Conference on Human Factors in Computing Systems, pp. 521–530 (2012). https://doi.org/10.1145/2207676.2207749
40. Marquardt, G., Bueter, K., Motzek, T.: Impact of the design of the built environment on people with dementia: an evidence-based review. HERD Health Environ. Res. Des. J. **7**(1), 127–157 (2014)
41. Institute of Medicine (US): The future of disability in America. The National Academies Press (2007). https://doi.org/10.17226/11898
42. Ministry of Land, Infrastructure, Transport and Tourism: law for promoting smooth mobility for the elderly and disabled (barrier-free law). chrome-extension://efaidnbmnnnibpcajpcglclefindmkaj/ https://www.mlit.go.jp/sogoseisaku/barrierfree/content/001328863.pdf. https://www.mlit.go.jp/sogoseisaku/barrierfree/ (2006)
43. Center for Inclusive Design and Environmental Access: Inclusive Design Guidelines: New York City. New York City Mayor's Office for People with Disabilities (2018) https://www.nyc.gov/html/mopd/html/initiatives/idg.shtml

Chapter 2
Conceptualizing Assistive Devices for the Elderly and Persons with Disabilities: The Research and Development Process

Toshiaki Tanaka

Abstract Assistive and rehabilitative engineering is an interdisciplinary field integrating medicine, therapy, and engineering to promote the independence and social participation of older adults and individuals with disabilities. This chapter provides an overview of the development of assistive devices, considering the International Classification of Functioning, Disability, and Health (ICF). The ICF offers a comprehensive framework for evaluating health conditions and environmental factors. The development process involves user-centered design, focusing on older adults and persons with disabilities, interdisciplinary collaboration, and iterative improvements from prototyping to commercialization. Additionally, this chapter discusses development methodologies for health, medical, and welfare-related devices that incorporate inclusive and barrier-free design concepts, emphasizing living environments that fully accommodate older adults' and persons with disabilities' needs.

2.1 Introduction

Welfare and rehabilitation engineering is an interdisciplinary field that systematizes engineering approaches to support people with disabilities and older adults. Integrating knowledge from medicine, physical therapy, occupational therapy, ergonomics, mechanical engineering, and information technology, it aims to promote individual independence and social participation. This paper explores the background of welfare and rehabilitation engineering and its relationship with the International Classification of Functioning, Disability, and Health (ICF). It also examines the device prescription and development process in health and welfare,

T. Tanaka (✉)
Research Center for Advanced Science and Technology / Institute of Gerontology, The University of Tokyo, Tokyo, Japan
e-mail: t.tanaka@iog.u-tokyo.ac.jp; tanaka@bfp.rcast.u-tokyo.ac.jp

T. Tanaka (ed.), *Inclusive and Barrier-Free Designs for Rehabilitation Engineering*,
https://doi.org/10.1007/978-981-95-5783-7_2

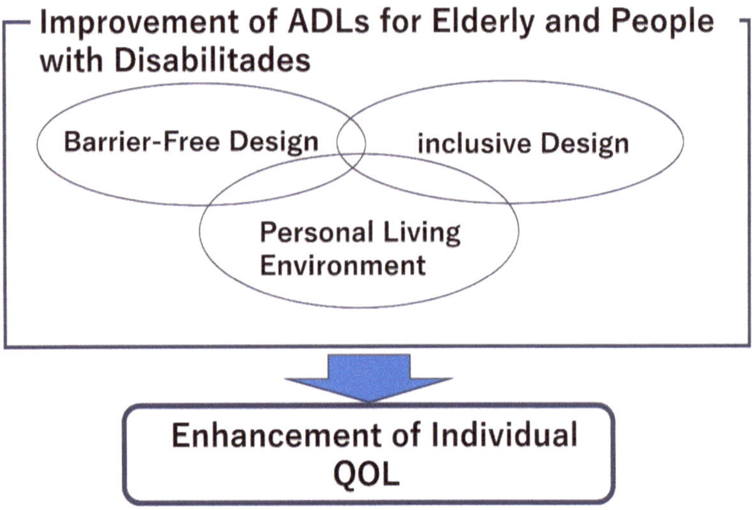

Fig. 2.1 Relationship between barrier-free/inclusive design and ADL/QOL

considering barrier-free and inclusive design. Finally, it discusses future prospects (Fig. 2.1).

2.2 Background and Relationship with ICF

Rehabilitation engineering advanced in the late 1970s, particularly in the United States, with a focus on assistive devices, such as prosthetics and orthotics [1]. In Japan, the Association of Rehabilitation Engineering was founded in 1986 to promote the dissemination of assistive technologies through medical-engineering collaboration. The theoretical foundation supporting this progress is the ICF, proposed by the World Health Organization (WHO) in 2001. The ICF provides a new framework for understanding disability from three perspectives: body functions and structures, activities, and participation. This framework enables a comprehensive approach that considers individual health conditions, as well as social and environmental factors [2]. For instance, limitations in physical function (e.g., restricted range of motion) can be compensated for with orthoses; limitations in activities (e.g., difficulty walking) can be alleviated with mobility aids; and restrictions in social participation can be addressed with home modifications or vocational training [3]. Thus, the ICF model serves as an essential evaluation framework in the development and introduction of assistive devices.

2.3 Definition and Institutional Background of Assistive Devices

"Assistive devices" are tools that support the daily lives, learning, and employment of persons with disabilities and older adults. These tools include prostheses, wheelchairs, communication devices, and toileting aids [4]. According to ISO 9999, assistive devices are defined as "products used to prevent, compensate for, or overcome impairments, activity limitations, or participation restrictions." In Japan, the Welfare Equipment Law institutionally supports the development and dissemination of assistive devices, and many devices are covered under the long-term care insurance and disability certificate systems [5]. Internationally, terms such as "assistive technology" or "assistive products and technology" are used, and the International Classification of Functioning, Disability, and Health (ICF) positions such products as part of environmental factors.

2.4 Device Prescription and Development Process

Proper implementation of assistive devices requires thorough dialogue with users and families, needs assessment, and training on how to wear and use the devices. For users with severe physical or cognitive disabilities, a team evaluation by physical therapists (PTs), occupational therapists (OTs), speech-language pathologists (SLPs), and psychologists is particularly essential [6]. The device selection process includes decisions regarding off-the-shelf versus custom-made options, trial periods, and follow-up within a comprehensive support system. Since devices directly impact patients' quality of life, clinicians must scientifically evaluate the characteristics of the disability and the compatibility of the device. The development process generally follows these steps: identifying field needs, assessing technical feasibility, designing and evaluating prototypes, conducting field tests, and commercialization [7]. Field voices from patients, families, caregivers, and healthcare providers serve as the starting point. Figure 2.2 illustrates the process from identifying needs to commercialization, emphasizing the importance of user feedback and researcher evaluation in refining prototypes before transitioning to patent acquisition, industry collaboration, and productization. Applying the development process shown in Fig. 2.2 to a patient's wheelchair, issues such as "difficulty operating in narrow spaces" and "fatigue from sitting for long periods" are first identified in care settings or hospitals. Next, researchers analyze the problems and assess the need for features such as weight reduction and posture adjustment. As solutions, wheelchairs with smaller turning radii or posture adjustment mechanisms are designed and prototyped and then evaluated in actual usage environments. Finally, through patent acquisition and collaboration with industry, the wheelchair is commercialized and introduced to the market.

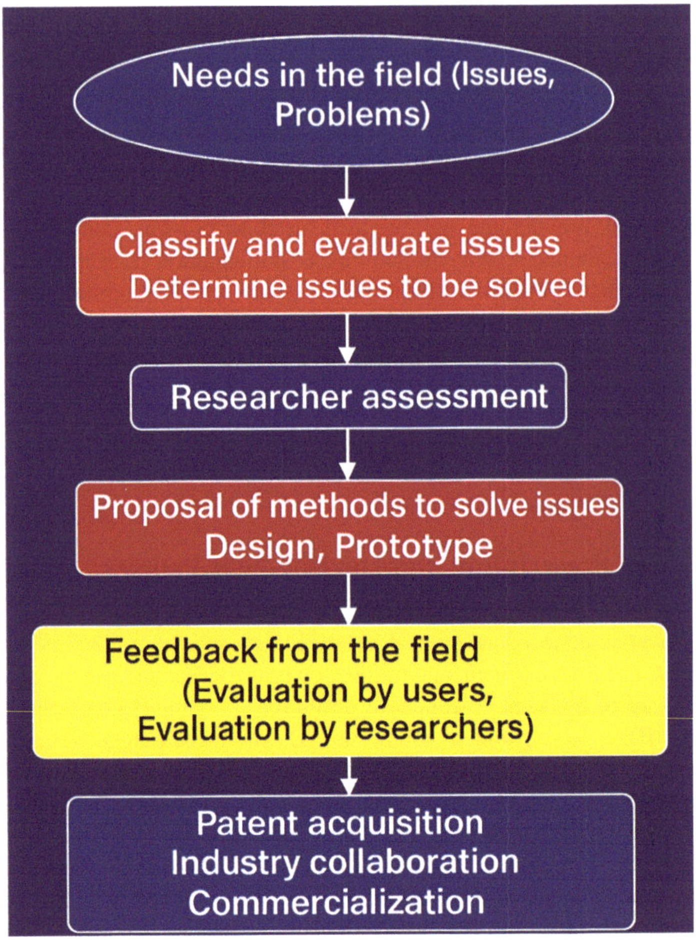

Fig. 2.2 Flow of development from needs to assistive device

Rehabilitation professionals, especially physical therapists (PTs) and occupational therapists (OTs), play a critical role as mediators because they have the closest contact with patients' daily lives. Understanding biomechanics, physiology, and ergonomics is essential to device design, while psychology, education, economics, distribution, and legal systems become critical during the dissemination stage [8].

2.5 Barrier-Free and Inclusive Design in Welfare Engineering

Recently, concepts such as universal design (UD) and inclusive design have gained importance in the design of assistive devices and environments. UD, which was popularized by architect Ronald Mace in the 1980s, aims to create products and environments that are usable by as many people as possible from the beginning [8]. In contrast, inclusive design focuses on incorporating diverse stakeholders, including people with disabilities, into the design process, emphasizing participation and flexibility [9]. These approaches shift away from the traditional "special measures for persons with disabilities" toward building an inclusive society where everyone has equal access [2]. In Japan, the AT2ED project by the Nakamura Laboratory at the University of Tokyo is a prime example. Home modifications such as removing steps, installing adjustable shelves, and using light sensors enhance convenience for various populations, demonstrating the fusion of engineering and architectural design. Furthermore, the introduction of barrier-free and inclusive design transforms development methodologies by emphasizing "user-centered design" (UCD), which involves end users from early design stages [6]. System-level measures, including institutional design and dissemination policies, are also critical. Figures 2.3 and 2.4 illustrate developmental research on new assistive devices and a combined social science and rehabilitation engineering study framework, highlighting the process from needs identification to commercialization

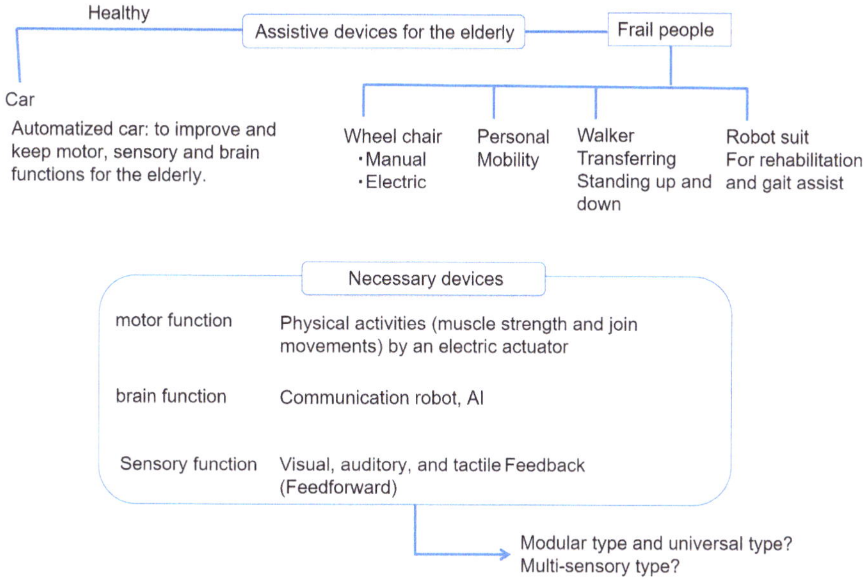

Fig. 2.3 Developmental research of new assistive devices for transferring of the elderly and disabled people

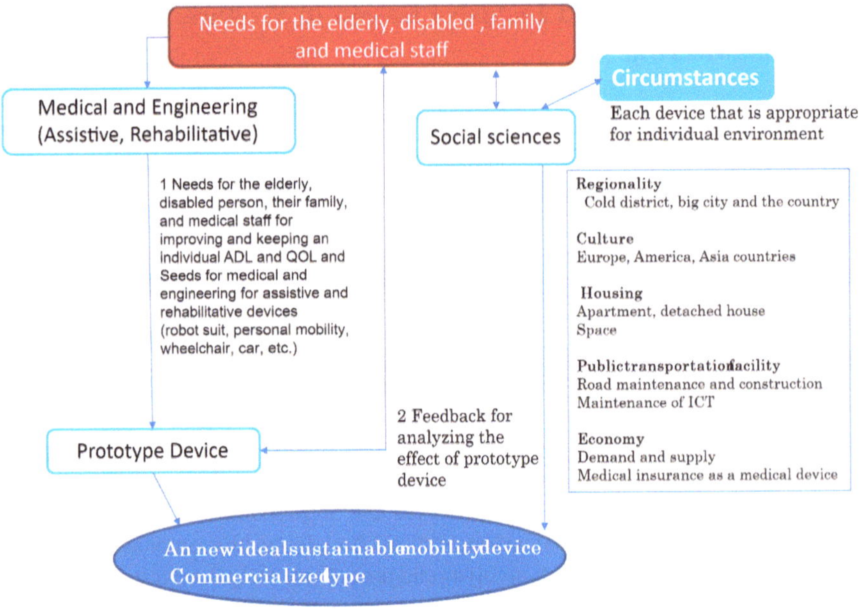

Fig. 2.4 A combined study of social science and rehabilitation engineering for developing assistive devices

[10]. Figure 2.3 explains developmental research on transfer support devices for elderly and frail individuals. The target population ranges from healthy elderly individuals to those who are frail. Appropriate assistive devices are presented for each stage. Mobility support devices include automated vehicles, wheelchairs (manual and electric), personal mobility devices, walkers, transfer aids, and rehabilitation robot suits, which are used according to an individual's physical and mental functional status, including motor, sensory, and cognitive functions. The ultimate goal is to develop versatile devices, such as modular or multi-sensory types, that can support the physical and mental functions of all elderly and disabled individuals. The development process of Fig. 2.4 can be explained using the example of a robotic suit that assists elderly individuals with gait disorders in walking. First, needs such as "fear of falling while walking" and "difficulty going out alone" are identified through input from the individuals, their families, and medical professionals. Medical and engineering professionals then develop prototypes of robotic suits to support muscle activity and degrees of freedom in the joints of the lower limbs. These suits assist with weakened muscle strength and joint impairments, which are necessary for standing up and climbing stairs. From a social science perspective, factors such as usability in cold climates, road conditions in urban and rural areas, cultural acceptance, and insurance coverage applicability are considered. Through evaluation and feedback based on real-world usage, the development and dissemination of an optimal robotic suit that enables elderly individuals to live independently in their communities are pursued.

2.6 Conclusion

Assistive and rehabilitative engineering plays a vital role in promoting social inclusion through technology. Based on personal experience in clinical settings, the author emphasizes that the needs of the field often drive innovation. Looking ahead, young rehabilitation professionals in Japan are expected to take the lead in connecting technology and welfare.

References

1. Cooper, R.A., Ohnabe, H., Hobson, D.A.: An Introduction to Rehabilitation Engineering. CRC Press (2006)
2. World Health Organization: International classification of functioning, disability and health (ICF). https://www.who.int/standards/classifications/international-classification-of-functioning-disability-and-health (2001)
3. Bauer, S.M., Elsaesser, L.-J., Arthanat, S.: Assistive technology device classification based upon the World Health Organization's, International Classification of Functioning, Disability and Health (ICF). Disabil. Rehabil. Assist. Technol. **6**(3), 243–259 (2011). https://doi.org/10.3109/17483107.2010.529631
4. Khasnabis, C., Heinicke Motsch, K., Achu, K., et al.: Community-Based Rehabilitation: CBR Guidelines. World Health Organization, Geneva (2010)
5. Ministry of Health, Labour and Welfare (MHLW): International classification of functioning—Revised international classification of impairments. https://www.mhlw.go.jp/houdou/2002/08/h0805-1.html (2002)
6. Cook, A.M., Polgar, J.M.: Assistive Technologies: Principles and Practice, 4th edn. Mosby (2015)
7. Federici, S., Scherer, M.J.: Assistive Technology Assessment Handbook. CRC Press (2018)
8. Mace, R.: Universal design in housing. Assist. Technol. **10**(1), 21–28 (1998). https://doi.org/10.1080/10400435.1998.10131957
9. Steinfeld, E., Maisel, J.: Universal Design: Creating Inclusive Environments. Wiley (2012)
10. Tanaka, T.: A study of new technologies of personal mobility and robot suit for the elderly and persons with disabilities. Fondation France-Japon de l'EHESS (CEAFJP DISCUSSION PAPER) #18-06 (18pages), 12 (2018)

Chapter 3
Supporting Individuals with Visual Impairments 1

Toshiaki Tanaka

Abstract For Sect. 3.1, unilateral spatial neglect (USN) is a common visual cognitive impairment after stroke that significantly limits activities of daily living (ADLs) and rehabilitation outcomes. Conventional assessments such as line cancellation, line bisection, and the Behavioral Inattention Test are clinically useful but often fail to capture real-world functional behavior. Rehabilitation methods including sensory stimulation, prism adaptation, and cognitive training have shown partial effectiveness, but recovery outcomes vary widely, underscoring the need for innovative strategies.

As described in Sect. 3.2, recent advances in virtual reality (VR) provide new opportunities for both assessment and intervention. Head-mounted display (HMD)-based studies have shown that visual field transformations and attentional cues can reveal spatial biases undetectable through paper-based tasks while improving patients' spatial exploration and attention redistribution. VR-based training promotes active participation, integrates multisensory feedback, and enhances visual-motor coordination, making it a promising approach for clinical rehabilitation.

With respect to Sect. 3.3, VR simulations are also emerging as powerful educational tools. By replicating conditions such as visual field constriction, cataracts, glaucoma, or lower limb weakness, VR enables learners—including healthcare students and caregivers—to directly experience disability-related challenges. This experiential approach fosters embodied empathy and strengthens awareness of supportive behaviors compared with traditional lectures. Postexperience reflection and group discussion further deepen understanding, in line with experiential learning theory.

Taken together, findings across Sects. 3.1, 3.2, and 3.3 demonstrate that VR plays a dual role in rehabilitation and education. Clinically, it offers immersive and patient-centered methods for evaluating and treating USN. Educationally, it cultivates empathy and disability awareness, helping prepare future professionals and caregivers for more effective and compassionate support. Future directions include

T. Tanaka (✉)
Research Center for Advanced Science and Technology/Institute of Gerontology, The University of Tokyo, Tokyo, Japan
e-mail: t.tanaka@iog.u-tokyo.ac.jp; tanaka@bfp.rcast.u-tokyo.ac.jp

T. Tanaka (ed.), *Inclusive and Barrier-Free Designs for Rehabilitation Engineering*,
https://doi.org/10.1007/978-981-95-5783-7_3

standardizing VR-based assessment and training protocols, expanding clinical trials, and designing structured educational frameworks to maximize its impact on inclusive and barrier-free rehabilitation practices.

3.1 Clinical Evaluation Methods and Current Rehabilitation of Visual Cognitive Impairment

Unilateral spatial neglect (USN) is one of the most frequently observed symptoms of visual perceptual disorders after stroke. USN typically occurs after brain damage, particularly in the right hemisphere, and involves neglecting one side of space or objects, especially the left side [1]. USN affects multiple sensory modalities, including vision, hearing, and touch. It causes issues in daily life, such as leaving food uneaten on the left side of the plate, forgetting to dress the left side of the body, or not responding to calls from the left.

USN is not merely a sensory disorder; it is classified as a higher brain dysfunction related to attention, cognition, and action. USN significantly affects functional independence, making early evaluation and intervention essential. Clinically, paper-and-pencil tests are primarily used for evaluation. Representative methods include the line cancellation test, star cancellation test, and line bisection test [2, 3]. In the line cancellation test, subjects are instructed to find and cross out lines that are randomly distributed on a sheet of paper. Omissions on the neglected side (typically the left) are an indicator of USN. In the line bisection test, subjects are asked to bisect horizontal lines on a page visually, but patients with USN tend to bisect lines toward the right. Copying and reading tasks, as well as the Behavioral Inattention Test (BIT), are also widely used [4].

Current rehabilitation methods are diverse and include sensory stimulation, behavioral therapy, cognitive training, and environmental adjustments. Among sensory stimulation techniques, visual scanning training is representative. This training repeatedly directs patients' attention to the neglected side to reduce neglect. Interventions that use nonvisual sensory modalities, such as cold water stimulation, vibratory stimulation, and electrical stimulation, are said to promote arousal of the neglected side [5].

Prism adaptation therapy has attracted attention in behavioral therapy. Wearing prism glasses facilitates adaptation to the visual space and improves attention toward the neglected side [6]. Cognitive training uses a metacognitive approach that encourages patients to recognize their symptoms of neglect and use attentional strategies. However, rehabilitation outcomes vary widely among patients, and individual differences exist in symptom recovery. Previous studies have identified predictive factors for recovery, including age, lesion location, time since onset, and initial neglect severity [7].

Furthermore, since USN has long-term effects on activities of daily living (ADLs) and quality of life (QOL), rehabilitation goals are not only limited to reducing symptoms but also include improving daily functioning and promoting social participation. Recently, new technological approaches have gained attention. These include virtual reality and robotics rehabilitation, as well as multisensory feedback methods that incorporate sensory integration. These approaches provide more immersive and motivating interventions than conventional methods [8].

Advancements in tele-rehabilitation technology have made it possible to provide continuous training at home, raising expectations for reducing disparities between regions and facilities. Thus, USN is a key target in the rehabilitation of visual perceptual disorders, and efforts are being made to promote patient independence and social participation through advances in clinical evaluation and intervention techniques. However, challenges remain, such as establishing standardized intervention methods, objectively evaluating intervention effects, and researching long-term outcomes. Continued development in these areas is required.

3.2 Development of Rehabilitation Device for Visual Cognitive Impairment

3.2.1 Introduction

Unilateral spatial neglect (USN) is a type of visual cognitive impairment that occurs following unilateral cerebral damage, such as a stroke. Patients with this condition ignore one side of their body or surrounding space. USN significantly limits activities of daily living (ADLs) and greatly affects rehabilitation outcomes [9, 10]. The pathology of USN is often understood through differences in spatial reference frames, which require evaluation from both egocentric and allocentric perspectives. Egocentric coordinate systems are based on the body (e.g., head, eyes, torso), while allocentric coordinates are based on the object itself. Impairments in these coordinate systems can result in the neglect of parts of objects or inattention to the left side of the body, thus influencing rehabilitation strategies [11]. Traditional clinical evaluations have relied heavily on paper-based tasks, such as the Behavioral Inattention Test (BIT), to evaluate the severity of USN through visual search, line bisection, and figure copying tasks [4]. However, these evaluations have limitations due to discrepancies with real-life behavior. Conversely, the Catherine Bergego Scale (CBS) evaluates neglect symptoms through observational assessments during daily activities. The CBS was developed to improve the reliability of clinical behavioral evaluations [12]. With advances in VR technology, more realistic evaluations and training have become possible. Studies by Tanaka et al. analyzed the effects of visual field transformation and visual stimulation using HMDs on patients' visual cognitive behavior, contributing to more sophisticated clinical assessments in Fig. 3.1 [13, 14].

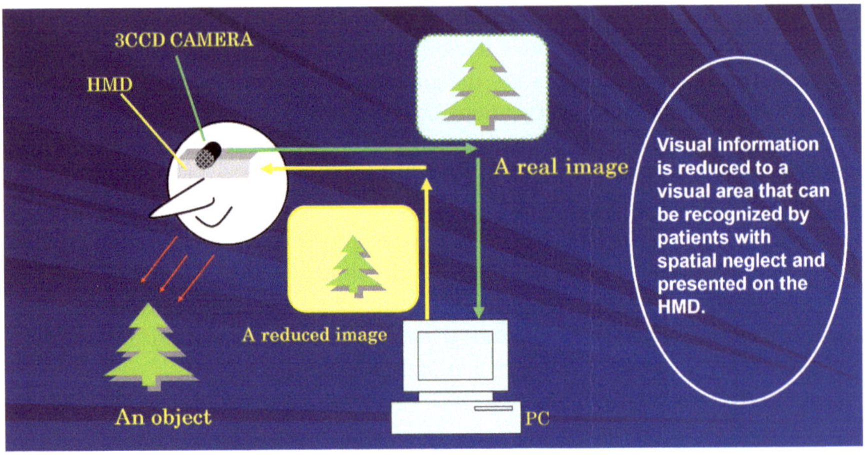

Fig. 3.1 Concept of the HMD system

3.2.2 Purpose

The purpose of this study is to clarify the effects of USN evaluations and training using a visual presentation system with an HMD. Specifically, we aimed to verify the impact of visual field enlargement/reduction and visual attention stimuli (arrow indicators) on spatial exploration behavior and compare their effectiveness to that of conventional paper-based evaluations.

3.2.3 Methods

The referenced studies [13, 14] used HMDs and charge-coupled device (CCD) cameras to create six visual presentation conditions based on egocentric and object-centered coordinate systems. Line cancellation tasks were conducted under each condition and included visual field resizing as well as flashing arrow stimuli on the left side (Fig. 3.2). Subjects included stroke patients diagnosed with USN. In addition to standard assessments using the BIT and CBS, visual field tasks using an HMD were employed to quantitatively evaluate left and right visual field omission rates.

3.2.4 Results

Although the BIT showed high scores in both visual fields, it was confirmed that the erasure rate in the left visual field was significantly lower when the visual field was

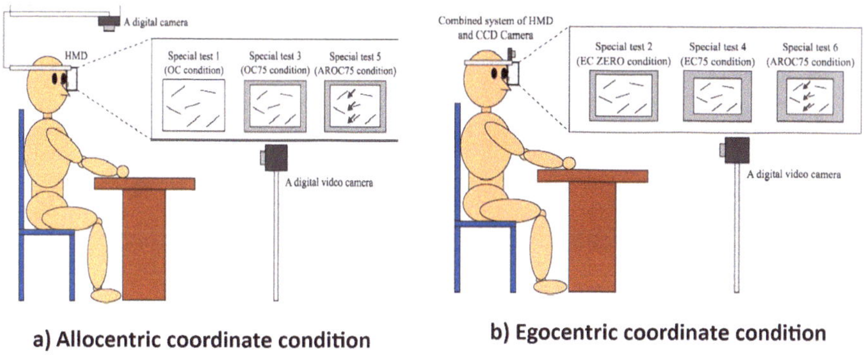

Fig. 3.2 Experimental setup for special tests (Allocentric coordinates and Egocentric coordinate condition) using the HMD combined system

presented under HMD conditions [13]. In particular, recognition accuracy on the left side was significantly reduced under the object-centered coordinate condition. However, an improvement trend was observed under the attention-grabbing arrow visual stimulation condition [14]. Patient A, who has a typical case of USN, improved his correct answers on the left side to 44% under the object-centered coordinates (OC) condition, 61% under the egocentric coordinates (EC) condition, and 72% with arrow stimulation. Conversely, Patient B, who also has USN, showed significant improvement with reduced visual field and arrow stimulation.

3.2.5 Discussion

This study shows that HMD-based visual field transformation and visual attention cues can visualize spatial biases in USN that are undetectable through paper-based assessments. We further evaluated depth perception and spatial cognition through object elimination tasks in a 3D virtual space. The authors reported the effectiveness of gaze guidance and attention cues during activities of daily living (ADLs) (Fig. 3.3) [15]. Ogourtsova et al. demonstrated that training with visual and sensory feedback effectively improves USN, which supports the effectiveness of visual stimulation observed in this study [16]. Kim et al. showed that switching between egocentric and allocentric coordinate systems in VR improves spatial exploration, which is consistent with the attention redistribution observed here. VR-based training encourages active participation and promotes visual-motor coordination through integrated sensory input [17]. Tanaka et al. evaluated neglect tendencies in walking and daily tasks within 3D environments and showed that virtual space feedback is effective for attention redistribution in Figs. 3.3 and 3.4 [18]. To clarify the mechanisms of rehabilitation and attention redistribution, analyzing brain activity is

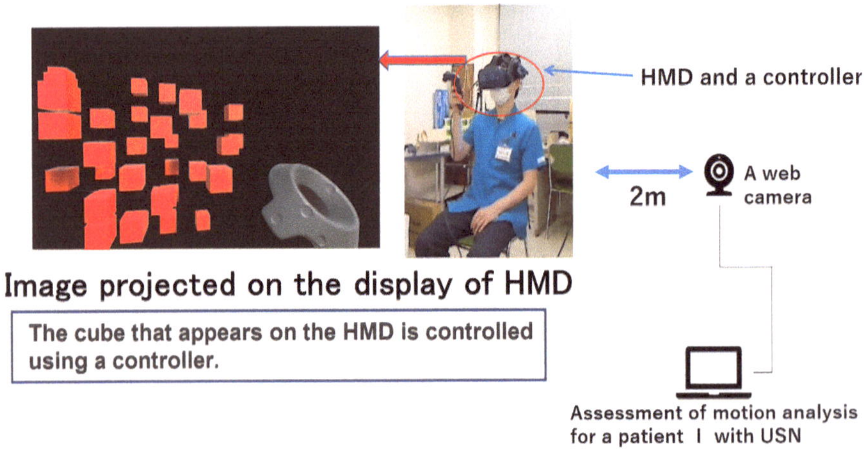

Fig. 3.3 Experiment setup for evaluation of USN by use of new HMD system

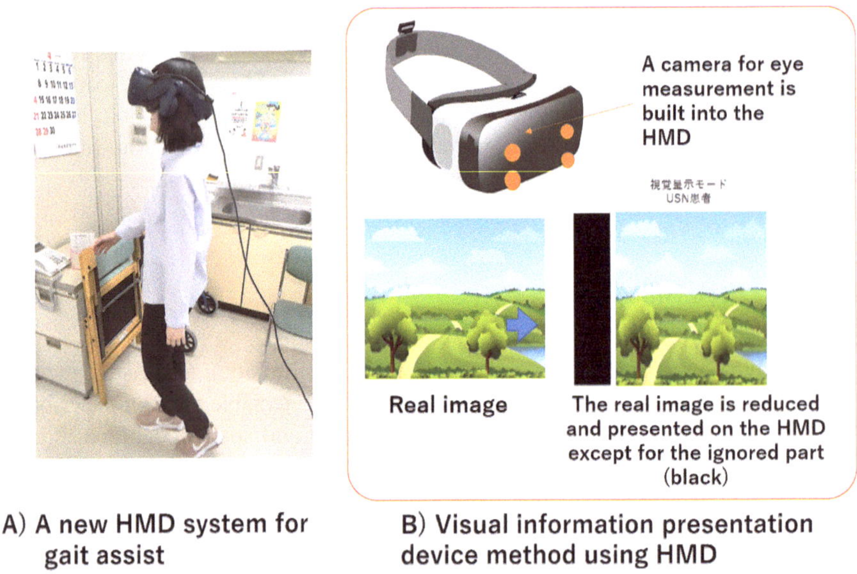

Fig. 3.4 Gait support using a 3D HMD system and a new method for displaying HMD images

essential. Recent studies using near-infrared spectroscopy (NIRS) and functional magnetic resonance imaging (fMRI) have visualized neural plasticity and activity changes in USN patients during training (Molenberghs et al.) [19], contributing to the design of tailored evaluations and training programs.

3.2.6 Conclusion

HMD-based USN evaluation and training methods are more effective than paper-based tasks at detecting and correcting spatial attention bias. This makes them promising for future clinical rehabilitation applications. Future developments should include broader participant samples and 3D task environments to facilitate more practical intervention design. Furthermore, as part of inclusive design research related to this study, this chapter introduced barrier-free research related to assistive devices for the assessment and training of individuals with visual cognitive impairments. In such cases, it is often difficult for others to fully understand how patients perceive their visual information. Therefore, opinions from patients themselves, as well as input from family members and medical staff involved in patient care, become critically important. In this context, the use of VR technology has enabled the simulation of a patient's spatial neglect, allowing the patient, family members, and medical staff to gradually gain understanding through a head-mounted display (HMD). If this HMD system can simulate environments that consider the home, outdoor settings, and regional characteristics, it is expected that such developments will expand into inclusive design research aimed at improving and enhancing patients' desired activities of daily living (ADLs) and quality of life (QOL).

3.3 Application of VR Visual Simulation as an Educational Tool

3.3.1 Introduction

In developed countries, including Japan, the population is aging rapidly, creating an increased demand for empathetic responses to the needs of the elderly and people with disabilities in medical and welfare settings. One significant impairment that severely affects daily living and poses a major rehabilitation issue is unilateral spatial neglect (USN), which is often observed after stroke. However, it is difficult for even medical staff and family members to understand how patients with USN perceive their environment or grasp the nature of their impairments. Training has been limited in its ability to reflect the challenges patients face in real-life contexts. Recently, VR has gained attention for its use in evaluating and training USN, allowing for more practical approaches through the realistic reproduction of spatial cognitive tasks and visual stimuli [20]. Similarly, educational institutions have begun introducing VR applications that simulate conditions such as narrowed visual fields, cataracts, glaucoma, and lower limb weakness—common disabilities in the elderly and patients. These applications provide learners with a sensory understanding that cannot be obtained through textbooks alone and are expected to foster a deeper understanding through embodied empathy [21, 22].

3.3.2 Methods

This study aimed to explore the utilization of VR-based simulations of sensory and motor impairments as educational tools. Specifically, we focused on (1) analyzing the design and characteristics of VR applications that simulate aging and visual impairments and (2) examining the application of VR in educational settings and its educational impact.

We developed a prototype VR application for education by combining a head-mounted display (HMD) with position sensors. This enables users to experience conditions such as age-related visual impairments, motor function decline, and USN poststroke subjectively. The app includes modes that simulate narrowing of the visual field, blurred vision similar to that caused by cataracts, and spatial neglect. It also allows for the simulation of lower limb impairment. Participants wearing the HMD can operate an actual wheelchair in a virtual environment while their motion data is analyzed. Each simulated experience can be adjusted to represent varying levels of severity (Figs. 3.5, 3.6, and 3.7).

3.3.3 Results

The VR simulation was designed so that participants could experience visual and physical limitations subjectively, allowing them to understand the difficulties faced by elderly individuals and people with disabilities physically and emotionally. Experience modes included blurred vision caused by cataracts, peripheral vision loss due to glaucoma, difficulty climbing stairs due to muscle weakness or sensory

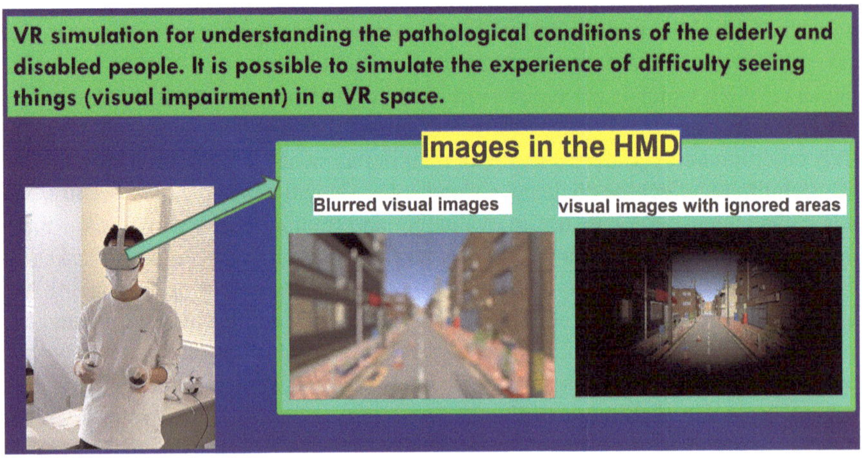

Fig. 3.5 Visual impairment experience by VR simulation

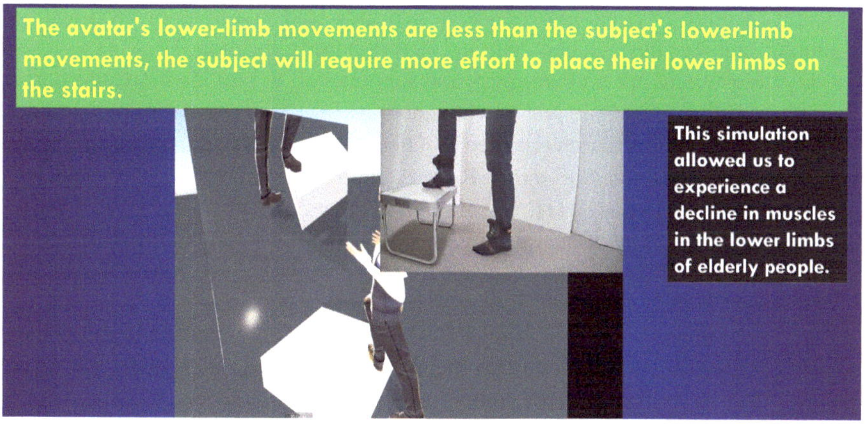
The avatar's lower-limb movements are less than the subject's lower-limb movements, the subject will require more effort to place their lower limbs on the stairs.
This simulation allowed us to experience a decline in muscles in the lower limbs of elderly people.

Fig. 3.6 Elderly experience VR simulation of ascending and descending stairs

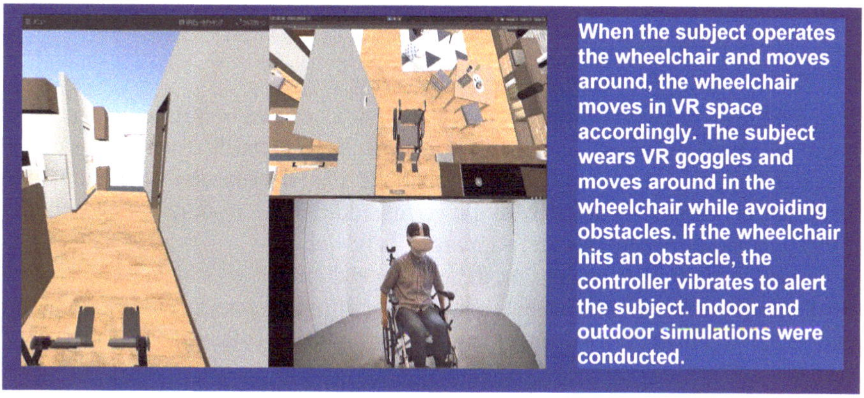

Fig. 3.7 Wheelchair operation experience by VR simulation

decline, and analysis of wheelchair maneuvering in various indoor and outdoor environments (Figs. 3.1, 3.2, and 3.3).

In practical educational settings, students were observed internalizing the concept of disability through direct experience, which led to a deeper understanding during postexperience reflection and group discussion. Classes that incorporated VR experiences showed a marked increase in students' awareness of supportive behaviors compared to traditional lectures [21, 23].

3.3.4 Discussion

The results suggest that VR visual simulation is more than just a tool for evaluation and training; it has significant educational value. Notably, it cultivates embodied empathy through physical experience, which may lead to a level of deep learning difficult to achieve through conventional lecture-based education. These experiences can lay the groundwork for caregivers and support staff to provide more appropriate and thoughtful assistance in real-world situations.

O'Connor et al.'s research reported that healthcare students gained cognitive and emotional understanding through VR-based aging simulations, further validating VR's educational impact [21]. Additionally, Herrera et al.'s study on empathy training using VR showed that such experiences can lead to long-term changes in supportive behavior [23].

To ensure educational effectiveness, programs should include reflection and group work immediately following the VR experience, in line with experiential learning theory. According to Kolb's theory [24], reflection on experience is essential for deep learning, and providing structural support is an effective way to maximize the educational impact of VR.

3.3.5 Conclusion

Based on prior research on USN rehabilitation and analysis of VR applications that simulate aging and visual impairments, this study has clarified the utility of VR visual simulation as an educational tool. VR experiences can elicit embodied empathy in learners and serve as powerful educational resources that promote understanding of disabilities and supportive behaviors.

Future tasks include comparing the educational effects across professions, standardizing the educational content, and developing indicators to evaluate learning outcomes. Additionally, we anticipate interdisciplinary collaborations with fields such as welfare, psychology, and engineering, as well as deployment in online learning environments.

References

1. Heilman K M, Valenstein E, Watson R T. Localization of neglect. In: Kertesz A, ed. Localization in Neurology New York: Academic Press. (1983)
2. Albert, M.L.: A simple test of visual neglect. Neurology. **23**(6), 658–664 (1973)
3. Halligan, P.W., Cockburn, J., Wilson, B.A.: The behavioural assessment of visual neglect. Neuropsychol. Rehabil. **1**(1), 5–32 (1991)
4. Wilson, B., Cockburn, J., Halligan, P. Development of a behavioral test of visuospatial neglect. Arch Phys Med Rehabil 68, 98–102. (1987)
5. Robertson, I.H., North, N.: Spatiomotor cueing in unilateral left neglect: therapeutic use and theoretical implications. Neuropsychologia. **30**(11), 979–988 (1992)
6. Rossetti, Y., Rode, G., Pisella, L., Farné, A., Li, L., Boisson, D., Perenin, M.T.: Prism adaptation to a rightward optical deviation rehabilitates left hemispatial neglect. Nature. **395**(6698), 166–169 (1998)

7. Katz, N., Hartman-Maeir, A., Ring, H., Soroker, N.: Functional disability and rehabilitation outcome in right hemisphere damaged patients with and without unilateral spatial neglect. Arch. Phys. Med. Rehabil. **80**(4), 379–384 (1999)
8. Tsirlin, I., Ring, H.: Virtual reality in neurorehabilitation of spatial neglect: a systematic review. NeuroRehabilitation. **29**(4), 305–318 (2011)
9. Heilman, K.M., Watson, R.T., Valenstein, E.: Neglect and related disorders. In: Clinical Neuropsychology. 2nd Edition, Oxford University Press, New York. (1985)
10. Bowen, A., et al.: Rehabilitation for spatial neglect in stroke patients. Cochrane Database. (1999)
11. Hillis, A.E., Rorden, C., Fridriksson, J.: Brain regions essential for resolving lexical ambiguity. Brain. **128**(4), 915–924 (2005)
12. Azouvi, P., et al.: Functional consequences and awareness of unilateral neglect: study of an evaluation scale. Neuropsychol. Rehabil. **13**(1–2), 133–145 (2003)
13. Tanaka, T., Sugihara, S., Nara, H., Ino, S., Ifukube, T.: A preliminary study of clinical assessment of left USN using HMD. J. Neuroeng. Rehabil. **2**, 31 (2005). https://doi.org/10.1186/1743-0003-2-31
14. Tanaka, T., Ifukube, T., Sugihara, S., Izumi, T.: A case study of new assessment and training of USN using HMD. J. Neuroeng. Rehabil. **7**, 20 (2010). https://doi.org/10.1186/1743-0003-7-20
15. Kudo, A., Kato, N., Miura, T., Tanaka, T.: Preliminary study on head and eye movements in patients with spatial neglect in different spatial domains using a head-mounted display. Pract. Sci. Occup. Ther. Jpn. **7**(2), 32–41 (2025). https://doi.org/10.32151/psot.7.2_32
16. Ogourtsova, T., Archambault, P.S., Lamontagne, A.: Post-stroke unilateral spatial neglect: a review of spatial and temporal factors and the effect of active interventions. Top. Stroke Rehabil. **25**(3), 187–199 (2018)
17. Kim, H., et al.: Egocentric vs. Allocentric neglect in immersive VR environments. Neuropsychologia. **155**, 107819 (2021)
18. Tanaka, T., Kato, N., Yagi, M., Hashimoto, N., Kudo, A., Sugihara, S.: Preliminary study on the assessment of patients with impaired visuospatial ability in three-dimensional space using a new head mounted display system with virtual reality technology. Int. J. New Technol. Res. **7**(4), 63–68 (2021). https://doi.org/10.31871/IJNTR.7.8.13
19. Molenberghs, P., Cunnington, R., Mattingley, J.B.: Brain regions with mirror properties: a meta-analysis of 125 human fMRI studies. Neurosci. Biobehav. Rev. **36**(1), 341–349 (2012)
20. Keller, I., Lefin-Rank, G.: Improved detection of neglect after visual cueing in VR. Neuropsychologia. **43**(1), 31–39 (2005)
21. O'Connor, M., Andreasen, J.: Enhancing empathy in medical students using VR-based aging simulations. J. Med. Educat. Curri. Develop. **7**, 238212052091660 (2020)
22. Dyer, M.L., et al.: Virtual reality and empathy: a meta-analysis. Front. Psychol. **9**, 2032 (2018)
23. Herrera, F., Bailenson, J.N., et al.: Building long-term empathy: a virtual reality intervention. PLoS One. **13**(10), e0204494 (2018)
24. Kolb, D.A.: Experiential Learning: Experience as the Source of Learning and Development, 2nd Edition, Pearson Education, Inc. (2015)

Chapter 4
Supporting Individuals with Visual Impairments 2: Walking and Navigating Support

Takahiro Miura and Toshiaki Tanaka

Abstract This chapter examines walking and navigation support systems for individuals with visual impairments, emphasizing sensory substitution functionalities and emerging assistive technologies. Worldwide, approximately 2.2 billion individuals are affected by vision loss. This chapter specifically emphasizes the distinctive perceptual abilities cultivated by individuals with visual impairments, including orientation and mobility (O&M), sound localization, obstacle detection via reflected sound, rapid comprehension of speech through screen readers, and tactile information derived from braille and tactile displays. Training methods include O&M instruction, acoustic virtual reality tools, and tactile maps created with specialized displays. Current navigation aids involve smartphone screen readers, outdoor mobility apps, indoor positioning systems, and AI-based visual recognition services. Despite technological advances, challenges in device use and access to training remain. Combining traditional mobility training with modern assistive technology offers a promising approach to enhancing independence and spatial awareness, both indoors and outdoors, for individuals with visual impairments.

4.1 Introduction

According to the World Health Organization, approximately 2.2 billion people worldwide have a vision impairment or blindness, with at least 1 billion of these cases being preventable or have yet to be addressed [1]. The leading causes of vision impairment globally are uncorrected refractive errors and cataracts, while the main

T. Miura
Research Institute on Human and Societal Augmentation (RIHSA), National Institute of Advanced Industrial Science and Technology (AIST), Chiba, Japan
e-mail: miura-t@aist.go.jp

T. Tanaka (✉)
Research Center for Advanced Science and Technology/Institute of Gerontology, The University of Tokyo, Tokyo, Japan
e-mail: t.tanaka@iog.u-tokyo.ac.jp; tanaka@bfp.rcast.u-tokyo.ac.jp

T. Tanaka (ed.), *Inclusive and Barrier-Free Designs for Rehabilitation Engineering*,
https://doi.org/10.1007/978-981-95-5783-7_4

causes of blindness include cataracts, glaucoma, age-related macular degeneration, and diabetic retinopathy [1]. Regionally, the highest prevalence of blindness occurs in sub-Saharan Africa and South Asia, with notable disparities between high- and low-income countries [2]. Similarly, vision impairment contributes to an estimated global economic burden of USD 411 billion annually [3]. This data highlights the urgent need for prevention, early detection, and appropriate intervention strategies worldwide.

As an example in Japan, there were 273,000 people with visual impairment as of 2022 [4]. The age distribution shows a clear skew toward older adults, with approximately 7000 people under the age of 20 years, 74,000 people aged 20–64 years, and 187,000 people aged 65 years or older [4]. This demographic pattern reflects the aging population in Japan and the increased prevalence of age-related eye diseases. The severity of visual impairment varied significantly by age group in 2016 but had become similar in 2022. In 2016, the percentage of those who have been certified as visually impaired at level 1 of class 1 (the most severe category) is 28.3% for those under 65 years and 42.3% for those aged 65 years or older in 2016 [4], but these percentages became 43.8% and 40.4% for those under and over 65 years, respectively [4]. The high percentage of older people with severe visual impairment in 2016 suggests that age-related diseases tend to progress to more advanced stages, while statistics from 2022 indicate that early detection may have improved among younger people. The main cause of visual impairment is reported to be congenital (birth) in 51.4% of children enrolled in special needs schools for the visually impaired, followed by retinopathy of prematurity (18.6%) and retinitis pigmentosa (13.9%) [5]. For all ages, glaucoma (28.6%), retinitis pigmentosa (14.0%), and diabetic retinopathy (12.8%) were reported to be the most common causes of visual impairments, in that order, and a similar trend was also observed in those aged 60 years and older [6].

Considering the significant global impact of visual impairment, support systems have undergone considerable improvement over the past two centuries. The first school for the blind in the world, the Royal Institute for Blind Youth (currently the National Institute for Blind Youth) in Paris, was established in 1784, and similar institutions later appeared throughout Europe and North America [7, 8]. Louis Braille's groundbreaking tactile reading system, introduced in 1824, fundamentally transformed literacy access for the visually impaired, laying the groundwork for modern assistive technologies [9, 10].

Modern legal frameworks include the Americans with Disabilities Act (1990), European Accessibility Act (2019), and the UN Convention on the Rights of Persons with Disabilities (2006), which established comprehensive civil rights protections and accessibility requirements. In Japan, formal education began during the Meiji period (1868–1912) with institutions like the Rakuzenkai Kunmouin blindness institute. Postwar legislation includes the Act on the Welfare of Persons with Disabilities (1949) and the Law for Eliminating Discrimination against Persons with Disabilities (2016), systematically addressing accessibility challenges [4, 11]. Modern assistive technologies include screen readers like NVDA

(NonVisual Desktop Access) and *VoiceOver*, supported by standardization efforts such as W3C WCAG 2.1.

As described above, the situation surrounding people with visual impairments is improving, but it is still in the development stage. This is because visually impaired individuals have unique sensory, perceptual, and cognitive systems [12–18]. Therefore, there is a challenge because methods of information transfer that work for sighted people are not always suitable for visually impaired individuals. By gaining a better understanding of these perception and recognition mechanisms, clinical practitioners, researchers, and developers can more effectively design and implement support systems and strategies to improve the capabilities of visually impaired people. This chapter discusses mobility and walking for individuals with visual impairments, highlighting their unique perceptual skills and support strategies.

4.2 Sensory Substitution Abilities in Visually Impaired Persons

Sensory substitution refers to the use of another sensory modality to alternatively acquire environmental information that is typically acquired by another sense [19, 20]. This subsection reviews research of sensory substitution reported in visually impaired persons.

4.2.1 Orientation and Mobility

In gait training, which is carried out for visually impaired persons to acquire independent mobility, the main focus is on orientation and mobility (O&M) [21, 22]. Orientation refers to environmental perception to know one's relative position in the surrounding environment, and mobility refers to physical mobility to move one's body in the direction of a destination. Practice and research on O&M abilities have been conducted with congenitally and acquired visually impaired individuals of various ages [23, 24]. There have been various studies on environmental perception by the visually impaired.

Orientation abilities include the localization of sound sources and non-sounding obstacles [25]. The localization performance of sound sources has been reported to vary depending on visual impairment status. Lessard et al. reported that the accuracy of horizontal directional localization in the blind was similar to that of the sighted, while the accuracy was lower in low-vision persons than in sighted persons [26]. Zwiers et al. reported similar results but also showed that in the vertical direction, the directional accuracy of sound source localization was lower for blind than for sighted participants [27]. Muchnik et al. reported that some visually impaired persons have better directional accuracy than sighted persons for horizontal

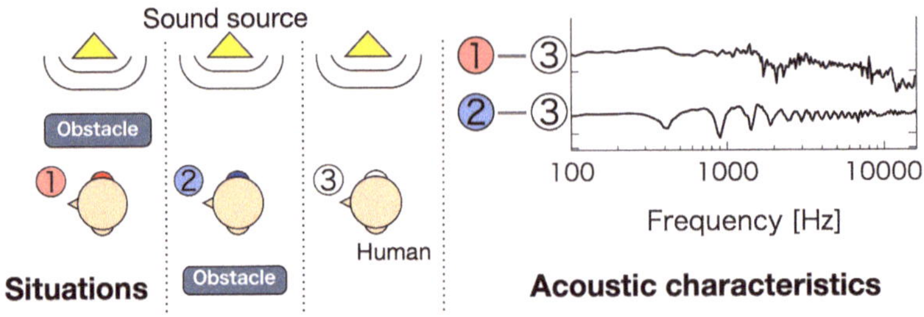

Fig. 4.1 Acoustic change caused by the presence of an obstacle [38]

sound source localization [28]. Therefore, it is possible that horizontal source localization accuracy can be improved without visual information, whereas visual experience may be important for vertical localization.

Regarding the localization of non-sounding obstacles, obstacle sense is one of the auditory spatial perceptual abilities that some blind people have acquired while the sighted have not. Obstacle sense is the ability to perceive the presence of a non-sounding object that itself emits no sound as a kind of discomfort or pressure feeling. The earliest description of the existence of this ability is given by Diderot in his *Letter on the Blind* (1749) [29]. As for the perceptual factors of obstacle sense, Heller et al. experimentally confirmed whether the cue for obstacle perception was cutaneous or auditory and confirmed that auditory perception was important [30]. Supa et al. conducted a similar study and reproduced the result that ear stimulation was the main factor [31]. Worchel et al. conducted a similar experiment with individuals with multiple audiovisual impairments and found that auditory stimulation, not stimulation of the external ear, was the main factor of the obstacle sense [32]. Cotzin et al. reported that reflected sound from an obstacle is important for the perception of the presence of an obstacle [33]. Regarding this reflected sound, Seki et al. experimentally confirmed the importance of coloration caused by the interference between the reflected sound and the background sound [34]. They experimentally confirmed the acoustic change of background sound caused by shielding, which has been called *sound shadows* [35–37], and reported its possible contribution to obstacle perception. Moreover, Miura et al. reported that components of the frequency band above 1 kHz in the gain and coloration changes associated with the presence of an obstacle, as well as the interaural level difference in the same frequency band, could be acoustic cues for obstacle perception [38]. Figure 4.1 summarizes the recognizable acoustic changes associated with the presence of an obstacle.

While individual differences exist in visual impairment status, differences have also been observed in the ability of obstacle sense. Kellogg and Rice studied discrimination of distance, size, and material of obstacles and reported that some individuals could discriminate distance with greater accuracy than visual depth perception and that some could distinguish differences in material as well as hardness of material [39–41]. Factors reported to enhance this ability include the person's forward/backward/right/left movements [42] and head rotational

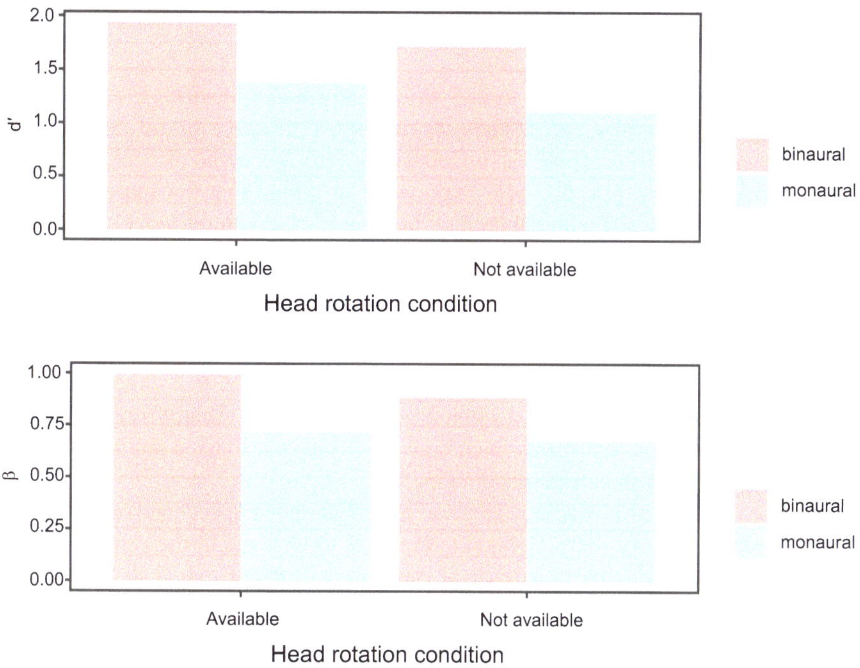

Fig. 4.2 Discrimination power d' (*upper*) and detection bias β (*lower*) with and without head rotation in binaural and monaural hearing [43]. The higher the d', the more accurately the presence of obstacles is recognized. β value close to 1.0 means that responses are unbiased, while a value less than 1.0 means that responses tend to indicate the presence of obstacles even when none exist

movements [43, 44] in response to obstacles, footsteps and the sound of a white cane [45, 46], and tongue-clapping behavior [47, 48]. Seki et al. showed that the preceding sound effect [49] may contribute to obstacle perception when a visually impaired person approaches an obstacle only when the obstacle is in close proximity [50]. Some of these experimental investigations were conducted with blindfolded sighted participants, and it has been shown that the presence of an obstacle can be perceived after a certain amount of training time [47, 51]. Miura et al. reported that head rotation and binaural hearing help accurately recognize obstacles and that when these are absent, responses biased toward indicating an obstacle may occur from a risk avoidance perspective (Fig. 4.2) [43]. Nakamura-Funaba et al. conducted a questionnaire survey among visually impaired people regarding the use of sound to support mobility and found some individual differences in the use of environmental sounds by visually impaired people, the ability to obtain more information from sounds through gait training, and difficulties in the use of sound by older visually impaired people [52]. Thus, it is presumed that obstacle sense can be acquired later in life, but it is more difficult in older age.

4.2.2 Perception of High-Speed Speech

To enable the visually impaired to use various information devices, a screen reader function has been implemented. The user can adjust the speed of the screen reader. Some visually impaired people can understand speech at a speed difficult for sighted people to understand [14, 53, 54]. Asakawa et al. found that the speed of speech understanding increased with habituation to the use of screen readers [14, 53]. Specifically, visually impaired subjects who had used screen readers for more than 5 years had a speech rate of approximately 1400–1500 mora/minute, and those who had never used a screen reader had a rate of approximately 60% when they repeated listening to a speech at approximately 1000–1150 mora/minute. The maximum reading speed of commercial screen readers at that time was about 878 mora/minute (designed by a sighted person), and the visually impaired could read much faster than this speed. Such high speeds have also been reported by users of English and Korean screen readers [55, 56].

The acquisition of obstacle perception and high-speed speech perception is not due to a sharpening of the peripheral system but to changes in the central nervous system through the unique experience of visual impairment. Bross et al. reported that the hearing levels of the visually impaired were not different from those of the sighted [57], and Starlinger et al. showed no difference in the perception of loudness and frequency changes between the visually impaired and sighted [58]. Benedett et al. found no difference in the perception of various auditory resolutions between the visually impaired and the sighted [59], and Miura et al. also found no difference in the perception of coloration changes between the two groups [16]. These results suggest that no acuity in the peripheral system occurs, and future research should be conducted on the experiences that led to the acquisition of unique perceptual abilities.

4.2.3 Perception of Tactile Information

Visually impaired individuals can also recognize and interpret text and texture information through their sense of touch. Visual impairment leads to tactile enhancement through complex neuroplastic mechanisms, with research consistently showing measurable improvements in tactile acuity, spatial resolution, and temporal processing abilities. Consequently, braille letters and diagrams are mainly used to help blind people understand text and diagrams.

Enhancing tactile abilities in visually impaired people exemplifies cross-modal neuroplasticity. Goldreich and Kanics reported that an average blind person has the tactile acuity of a sighted person of the same gender who is 23 years younger, suggesting that cross-modal plasticity may contribute to enhanced tactile acuity in blindness [60]. Neuroimaging studies demonstrate that visual cortex areas are recruited for tactile processing, with distinct neural correlates for different tactile dimensions including rough/smooth, sticky/slippery, and soft/hard textures [12, 61]. This form of cross-modal plasticity improves spatial processing abilities, surpassing the performance of sighted people. The timing of visual impairment affects tactile development. Ahulló-Fuster et al. found different cortical remapping in those blind early versus late [62]. Particularly, early deprivation leads to greater tactile improvements, with blindness before age 5 causing more visual cortical reorganization for touch, while late blindness relies more on attention and strategies.

Concerning tactile performance, Van Boven et al. studied spatial resolution and found that blind braille readers had average discrimination thresholds of 1.04 mm, compared to 1.46 mm in sighted people [63]. The primary reading finger had a threshold of 0.80 mm, and even fingers not used for braille performed better than sighted individuals at 1.12 mm, indicating a broad tactile enhancement beyond specific training. Temporal resolution in visually impaired individuals also demonstrates remarkable precision, detecting pulse-to-vibration changes at 30 ms and processing frequencies up to 590 Hz through Pacinian receptors [64]. Regarding texture discrimination, Alary et al. reported the tactile abilities in both blind and sighted individuals [65]. Although there were no significant differences in grating orientation or vibrotactile frequency tasks, their results suggested that blind individuals performed better in texture discrimination—likely due to their familiarity with braille. This indicates that the braille reading experience may enhance specific tactile skills.

Braille, specifically six-dot braille, was developed by Louis Braille in 1824 and remains in use today [10]. The dot size of braille characters is approximately 0.5 mm, and the dot spacing typically ranges from 2.0 to 2.5 mm (width) and 3.0 to 4.0 mm (height), with some variation across countries [66]. Braille reading speed depends on disability status, age at onset, and training experience. Mutaguchi's study of 36 experienced readers found median speeds of 124 wpm, with Japanese Grade 1 (total blind and severe low vision) readers reading at 71.5% of Grade 2 (low vision), influenced by braille contractions and abbreviations that reduce cognitive load [67]. Regarding developmental improvement, McCarthy et al. found that elementary students (grades 1–2) read 16.80–18.37 words/min, and middle school students (grades 7–9) reach 45.82–50.51 words/min using refreshable braille [68]. Additionally, studies on expert adults indicate speeds of around 70–100 words/min [69], an average of 136 words/min (range: 65–185) [70], and between 60 and 300 words/min [71]. For Japanese, the Ministry of Education, Culture, Sports, Science and Technology (MEXT) describes 150 cells/min at the end of initial learning, 300 cells/min for standard subject learning, 450 cells/min for efficient learning, and an ideal rate of 600 cells/min [72]. Adult braille learning encounters difficulties with modest outcomes. Bola et al. found that sighted adults averaged only 6.20 words/min after training, highlighting critical period effects and limiters such as reduced tactile sensitivity, established visual reading habits, and decreased neuroplasticity compared to childhood [73].

4.3 Sensory Substitution Techniques to Aid Auditory Perception of Space and Training Methods

4.3.1 Supporting and Training of Orientation and Mobility

In O&M, various walking aids have been developed to support orientation (environmental perception) in real space. In particular, the primary focus has been on acquiring information that cannot be obtained sufficiently by a white cane or a guide dog, as visually impaired people learn to use such devices during the course of functional training for daily life. Representative examples of auditory sensory substitution devices include the spectacle-type Sonic Guide and the handheld Mowat Sensor [74, 75]. These methods utilize ultrasonic waves to measure the distance to an object and then convert it into an audible signal according to the distance.

The Sonic Guide presented distance in terms of sound level and direction as the difference between the two ears, and the Mowat Sensor presented vibrations and sounds with frequencies corresponding to the distance. Many similar systems have been developed, including those using ultrasonic waves to acquire environmental information (e.g., ultrasonic eyeglasses [76] and others [77], cameras, vOICe [78], and FingerReader2.0 [79]). Furthermore, a combination of a white cane and walking aids is listed as Ultra Cane using ultrasonic waves, K-Sonar cane [80], laser cane using a laser [81], and WeWalk, which links various sensors and functions of a smartphone [82]. However, even commercialized devices have not been easily proficient. In addition, due to delays in the development of training manuals in rehabilitation and educational settings and a lack of trainers who can provide instruction, the use of these devices has not become widespread, at least in Japan [15].

In the context of gait training, training methods for sound source localization and obstacle sense have been developed. Seki et al. developed a system that enables users to train in a simulated outdoor sound environment using acoustical virtual reality (VR) [83]. Furthermore, by combining real-world walking and acoustic VR in a safe and spacious environment, they developed a wide-range auditory orientation training system (WR-AOTS) [84] and then distributed it to schools for the visually impaired. Similar systems exist, such as one that mainly trains sound source localization ability [85, 86] and systems that present only the presence and distance of obstacles [87]. Additionally, based on the author's mini-interview with a blind person with extensive auditory experience, it was found that the external sound pass-through and personalized audiogram-based hearing compensation functions of headphones might be able to enhance the acoustic detection accuracy of approaching vehicles, ground structures, obstacles, and snow conditions by utilizing reflected sound and low-frequency components. However, high-intensity environmental noise and wind noise reduction processing were noted to attenuate critical acoustic cues, potentially decreasing detection performance.

4.3.2 Information Acquisition Support by Tactile Presentation

Numerous studies have been conducted to provide information on the development and use of tactile dot-matrix displays, along with the output of tactile maps and their applications.

Tactile maps are often used in educational and social contexts [88]. In educational settings, they are used for pictures for science, technology, engineering, and mathematics (STEM) or science, technology, engineering, art, and mathematics (STEAM) education, such as graphs and equations, braille books with images, electronic circuits, hypertext markup language (HTML) Web pages, images for computer science and physics, and VR objects. Meanwhile, the social life aspect includes traveling and tactile graphics, maps and audio guidance, artworks and objects' shape, haptic and braille display, and orientation and mobility contexts. For tactile map generation, *tmacs* developed by Watanabe et al. [89] is a good example in Japan; it can be used after map creation on a website and printed on capsule paper using specialized printers.

Large-scale pin-matrix displays are often used for tactile dot displays. DotView DV-1 and DV-2 (KGS) are available in Japan, and Graphiti (Orbit Research) and Dot Pad (Dot Inc.) are available internationally. Sakai et al. have proposed a tactile-proprioceptive (tactile-prop) display that guides the user to the position to be traced by merging with force sensation using Phantom [90, 91] (Fig. 4.3) and have used it to understand maps and the human body structure.

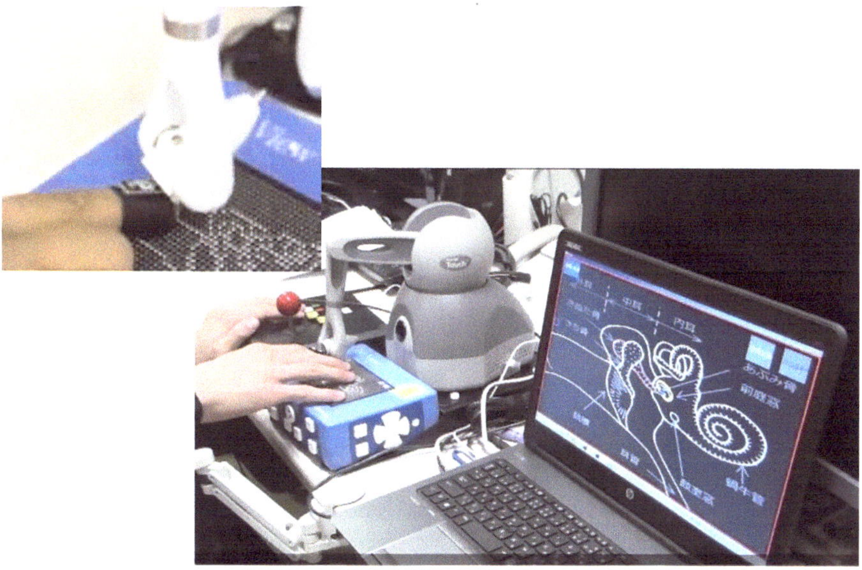

Fig. 4.3 Tactile-prop display that guides the user's finger with force using Phantom [90, 91]

Mobility support using vibrotactile body presentation provides real-time navigation guidance and obstacle detection. The *feelSpace belt* utilizes 13 vibrotactile motors around the waist and signals the magnetic north as a fixed reference frame via vibro-tactile stimulation [92]. After 7 weeks of training, blind participants reported increased confidence in navigation. Jeong and Yu developed a system integrating seven ultrasonic sensors with fingertip-mounted tactile displays, achieving 88.6% obstacle avoidance success rates [93]. Wersényi evaluated an eight-channel tactile feedback system with vibrators on wrists, arms, ankles, and forehead, finding that 2–4 channels can be used simultaneously with high accuracy, with optimal placement on wrists and signal duration exceeding 500 ms [94].

4.3.3 Navigation and Information Acquisition Support

In the last 20 years, screen readers that read aloud to visually impaired users for accessing graphical user interfaces (GUI) have been developed and improved, and many systems based on such readers have been implemented.

The pioneering Japanese-language GUI screen readers include *95Reader*, *PC-Talker*, and *focus talk*. A feature unique to the Japanese screen readers is the detailed reading (tamachi yomi) of kanji developed by Watanabe et al. [95]. This feature explains each kanji character one by one so that users can distinguish homonyms and synonyms. In addition to these screen readers, the free and highly functional NVDA, *Narrator* (Windows based), VoiceOver (macOS based), and *TalkBack* (Android based), which are included in the operating system preinstallation, are available in multiple languages. Screen readers are now commonplace for individuals with visual impairments. Moreover, speech reading has become more natural, and Imai et al., for example, have developed a method to further improve transmission efficiency by converting the speech speed for each character type [54]. Currently, the challenges are to extend the range of GUI access and improve the efficiency of operation under the use of screen readers. Asakawa et al. developed a homepage reader for accessing websites [96]. Next, they constructed tactile jog dial (*TAJODA*), which is a screen reader plus a tactile display, and achieved the cueing of various Web articles [14]. Furthermore, many other usability improvements of screen readers have been studied, including support for multimedia contents and efficient multitasking by a user's own efforts [97–99].

With the recent increase in the number of mobile devices, such as smartphones, there are more and more cases of screen reader-based real-world accessibility support. Kane et al. proposed the slide rule, a set of gestures for visually impaired users of touchscreen terminals, and it is now a standard specification for them to manipulate smartphones [101]. Based on these rules, an increasing number of systems have been developed to present navigation and map information, especially to the visually impaired. *Kotonavi* and *Navireco* are examples of outdoor mobility aids in Japan. Both systems use a screen reader to read out route guidance created on the Web. In addition, *BlindSquare* is well known for obtaining information on

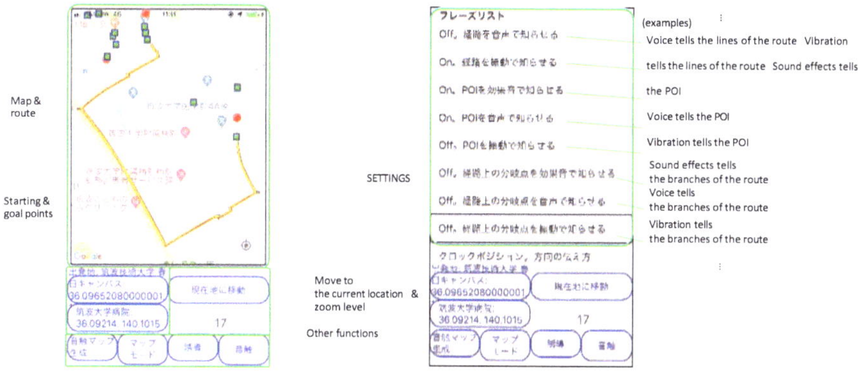

Fig. 4.4 (Left) Navigation view and (right) setting view for audio-tactile effects of *OTASCE Map* [100]

nearby facilities [102]. Indoor mobility support includes *NavCog*, which use self-positioning identification based on in-terminal sensors and (Bluetooth low energy) beacons [103, 104]. Matsuo et al. developed *OTASCE Map* (Oto-TActile SCapE Map) (Fig. 4.4), a route presentation application that can control voice, sound effects, and vibration to help visually impaired people understand route information in advance [100]. They investigated the preferred multimodal information when presenting routes to blind and low-vision people and found that it is desirable for blind people to be presented with all of sound, sound effect, and vibration and for low-vision people to be presented with one of sound, sound effect, or vibration as a supplement to visual information. They also found that visually impaired users prefer voice prompts before becoming proficient with the app but prefer sound effects as they become more proficient [105].

Other research includes the development of navigation robots for visually impaired individuals. Shoval et al. proposed *NavBelt and Guide-Cane* to assist outdoor walking [106], while Guerreiro et al. proposed Carry-on Robot (*CaBot*), an autonomous suitcase-type robot to assist indoor walking [107]. CaBot has been reported to be applied as a guide in museum exhibitions in the 2020s [108].

Systems have also been developed to assist the visually impaired in understanding visual information in the real world via remote volunteers and artificial intelligence. The *VizWiz* by Bicham et al. allows visually impaired people to take a picture of something they want to know and upload it together with a text question (visual question answering, VQA), and then a sighted volunteer on the Web provides the content of the picture in text form [109]. Similar systems, such as *Be My Eyes*, *TapTapSee*, and *CamFind*, have appeared [110], and VizWiz was later converted to a machine learning model by building a classifier that learned from the VQA dataset [111]. Seeing AI and Envision AI are also examples of similar systems that have utilized a machine learning model [112, 113]. There are increasing numbers of such systems that continue to be introduced and improved with the involvement of visually impaired users, and we can expect further developments in the future [114].

4.4 Conclusion

Fundamental to independent mobility is orientation and mobility (O&M) training for visually impaired individuals, which encompasses environmental perception for spatial awareness and physical movement skills. Research shows that visually impaired people develop improved auditory spatial perception, such as better sound source localization in horizontal directions and obstacle detection—the ability to sense non-sounding objects through reflected sound analysis. These skills depend on acoustic cues like sound coloration changes, sound shadows, and frequency components above 1 kHz, rather than on enhanced peripheral hearing sensitivity.

Technological sensory substitution has evolved from early ultrasonic devices, such as the Sonic Guide and Mowat Sensor, to advanced smartphone-based systems. Modern screen readers (NVDA, VoiceOver, TalkBack, and Narrator) provide access to digital information, with some users reaching comprehension speeds of 1400–1500 mora/min—much faster than normal speech rates. Tactile information processing through braille remains essential, with reading speeds ranging from 16.8 to 300 words/min influenced by visual conditions and individual braille experiences and supported by tactile displays and pin-matrix systems for spatial information.

Training methodologies have incorporated virtual reality environments, exemplified by the Wide-Range Auditory Orientation Training System (WR-AOTS), which combines real-world walking with acoustic simulation. Tactile map generation systems like tmacs enable spatial understanding through specialized printing technologies and large-scale pin-matrix displays.

Contemporary navigation support integrates multiple technological approaches. Outdoor mobility applications provide GPS-based navigation with speech synthesis, while indoor positioning systems like NavCog utilize sensor fusion and Bluetooth beacons for precise localization. AI-powered visual recognition services, including VizWiz, Be My Eyes, and Seeing AI, enable real-time environmental understanding through crowdsourced assistance and machine learning algorithms.

Despite remarkable technological advances, adoption challenges persist due to the complexity of training, high device costs, and limited rehabilitation infrastructure. Future developments must address these barriers while continuing to leverage the remarkable adaptive capabilities demonstrated by visually impaired individuals in spatial navigation and environmental perception.

References

1. World Health Organization, et al.: https://www.who.int/publications/i/item/world-report-on-vision, Last accessed 2025.12.18 (2019)
2. Bourne, R.R., Flaxman, S.R., Braithwaite, T., Cicinelli, M.V., Das, A., Jonas, J.B., Keeffe, J., Kempen, J.H., Leasher, J., Limburg, H., et al.: Lancet Glob. Health. **5**(9), e888 (2017)

3. Fricke, T.R., Tahhan, N., Resnikoff, S., Papas, E., Burnett, A., Ho, S.M., Naduvilath, T., Naidoo, K.S.: Ophthalmology. **125**(10), 1492 (2018)
4. Ministry of Health, Labour and Welfare, Japan. https://www.mhlw.go.jp/content/11704000/000955880.pdf (2022)
5. Kakizawa, T.: Jyakushi-Kyouiku. **49**(4), 6 (2012)
6. Morizane, Y., Morimoto, N., Fujiwara, A., Kawasaki, R., Yamashita, H., Ogura, Y., Shiraga, F.: Jpn. J. Ophthalmol. **63**, 26 (2019)
7. Koestler, F.A.: The Unseen Minority: A Social History of Blindness in the United States. American Foundation for the Blind. Arlington, Virginia, U.S. (2004)
8. French, K.: Perkins School for the Blind. Arcadia Publishing. Charleston, South Carolina, U.S. (2004)
9. Mellor, C.M.: Louis Braille: A Touch of Genius. National Braille Press. Boston, MA, U.S. (2006)
10. Jiménez, J., Olea, J., Torres, J., Alonso, I., Harder, D., Fischer, K.: Surv. Ophthalmol. **54**(1), 142 (2009)
11. Cabinet Office, Government of Japan: https://www8.cao.go.jp/shougai/suishin/jirei/
12. Sadato, N., Pascual-Leone, A., Grafman, J., Deiber, M.P., Ibanez, V., Hallett, M.: Brain J. Neurol. **121**(7), 1213 (1998)
13. Seki, Y.: J. Acoust. Soc. Jpn. **60**(6), 325 (2004)
14. Asakawa, C., Takagi, H., Ino, S., Ifukube, T.: IEICE Trans. Inf. Syst. **87**(6), 1405 (2004)
15. Ifukube, T.: Sound-Based Assistive Technology. Springer, Cham, Switzerland (2017)
16. Miura, T., Muraoka, T., Ifukube, T.: Acoust. Sci. Technol. **31**(2), 137 (2010)
17. Bach-y Rita, P., Kercel, S.W.: Trends Cogn. Sci. **7**(12), 541 (2003)
18. Chebat, D.R., Harrar, V., Kupers, R., Maidenbaum, S., Amedi, A., Ptito, M.: Mobility of Visually Impaired People: Fundamentals and ICT Assistive Technologies, pp. 167–200 (2018)
19. Bach-y Rita, P.: Acta Neurol. Scand. **43**(4), 417 (1967)
20. Bach-y Rita, P., Collins, C.C., Saunders, F.A., White, B., Scadden, L.: Nature. **221**, 963 (1969)
21. LaGrow, S.J., Weessies, M.J.: Orientation and Mobility: Techniques for Independence. Dunmore Press Palmerston North, New Zealand (1994)
22. Wiener, W.R., Welsh, R.L., Blasch, B.B.: Foundations of Orientation and Mobility, vol. 1. American Foundation for the Blind. Arlington, Virginia, U.S. (2010)
23. Ambrose, G.V.: J. Vis. Impair. Blind. **94**(8), 509 (2000)
24. Kuyk, T., Elliott, J.L., Wesley, J., Scilley, K., McIntosh, E., Mitchell, S., Owsley, C.: J. Rehabil. Res. Dev. **41** (2004)
25. Miura, T., et al.: Psychologia. **65**(1), 70 (2023)
26. Lessard, N., Paré, M., Lepore, F., Lassonde, M.: Nature. **395**(6699), 278 (1998)
27. Zwiers, M. P., van Opstal, A. J., & Cruysberg, J. R. M. (2001). A spatial hearing deficit in early-blind humans. The Journal of Neuroscience, 21(9), Article RC142. https://doi.org/10.1523/JNEUROSCI.21-09-j0002.2001
28. Muchnik, C., Efrati, M., Nemeth, E., Malin, M., Hildesheimer, M.: Scand. Audiol. **20**(1), 19 (1991)
29. Diderot, D.: In: Diderot, D., Adams, D.J. (eds.) Thoughts on the Interpretation of Nature and Other Philosophical Works. Clinamen Pr Ltd, Manchester, U.K. 2000 (1749)
30. Heller, T.: Studien zur Blinden-Psychologie. Wilhelm Engelmann (1904)
31. Supa, M., Cotzin, M., Dallenbach, K.M.: Am. J. Psychol. **57**(2), 133 (1944)
32. Worchel, P., Dallenbach, K.M.: Am. J. Psychol. **60**(4), 502 (1947)
33. Cotzin, M., Dallenbach, K.M.: Am. J. Psychol., 485–515 (1950)
34. Seki, Y., Ito, K.: IEEE Trans. Speech Audio Process. **11**(6), 817 (2003)
35. Wright, H.N.: Proc. Int. Congr. Technology and Blindness, pp. 149–157 (1963)
36. Welch, J.: Res. Bull. Am. Found. Blind. No. **4**, 1–13 (1964)
37. Kehler, I.: Res. Bull. Am. Found. Blind. **4**, 55 (1964)
38. Miura, T., Ifukube, T., Furukawa, S.: J. Acoust. Soc. Jpn. **67**(7), 261 (2011)
39. Kellogg, W.N.: Science. **137**(3528), 399 (1962)

40. Rice, C.E., Feinstein, S.H.: Science. **148**(3673), 1107 (1965)
41. Rice, C.E.: Science. **155**(3763), 656 (1967)
42. Rosenblum, L.D., Gordon, M.S., Jarquin, L.: Ecol. Psychol. **12**(3), 181 (2000)
43. Miura, T., Okochi, N., Suzuki, J., Ifukube, T.: Int. J. Environ. Res. Public Health. **20**(8), 5573 (2023)
44. Miura, T., Okochi, N., Matsuo, M., Yabu, K., Katagiri, A., Yasu, K., Sakajiri, M., Ifukube, T.: Life. **14**(3), 356 (2024)
45. Strelow, E.R., Brabyn, J.A.: Perception. **11**(6), 635 (1982)
46. Schenkman, B.N., Jansson, G.: Hum. Factors. **28**(5), 607 (1986)
47. Rojas, J.A.M., Hermosilla, J.A., Montero, R.S., Espí, P.L.L.: Acta Acust. united Acust. **95**(2), 325 (2009)
48. Thaler, L., Arnott, S.R., Goodale, M.A.: PLoS One. **6**(5), e20162 (2011)
49. Wallach, H., Newman, E.B., Rosenzweig, M.R.: J. Acoust. Soc. Am. **21**(4), 468 (1949)
50. Seki, Y., Ifukube, T., Tanaka, Y.: J. Acoust. Soc. Jpn. **50**(4), 289 (1994)
51. Ammons, C.H., Worchel, P., Dallenbach, K.M.: Am. J. Psychol. **66**(4), 519 (1953)
52. Nakamura-Funaba, H., Ueda, M., Iwamiya, S.: J. Acoust. Soc. Jpn. **62**(12), 839 (2006)
53. Asakawa, C., Takagi, H., Ino, S., Ifukube, T.: Proceedings of the 2003 International Conference on Auditory Display (ICAD 2003), pp. 276–279 (2003)
54. Imai, A., Tazawa, N., Takagi, T., Tanaka, T., Ifukube, T.: IEEE Trans. Consum. Electron. **59**(1), 200 (2013)
55. Moos, A., Trouvain, J.: Proceedings of the 16th International Congress of Phonetic Sciences, vol. 1, pp. 677–680. Saarland University, Saarbrücken (2007)
56. Lee, H., Jang, Y., Hong, K.H.: Computers Helping People with Special Needs: 14th International Conference, ICCHP 2014, Paris, France, July 9–11, 2014, Proceedings, Part I 14, pp. 49–52. Springer (2014)
57. Bross, M., Borenstein, M.: Percept. Mot. Skills. **55**(3), 963 (1982)
58. Starlinger, I., Niemeyer, W.: Audiology. **20**(6), 503 (1981)
59. Benedetti, L.H., Loeb, M.: Percept. Psychophys. **11**, 10 (1972)
60. Goldreich, D., Kanics, I.M.: J. Neurosci. **23**(8), 3439 (2003)
61. Kim, J.H., Kim, S.P.: Investig. Magn. Reson. Imaging. **27**(1), 1 (2023)
62. Ahulló-Fuster, M.A., Sánchez-Sánchez, M.L., Varela-Donoso, E., Ortiz, T.: PLoS One. **19**(7), e0306478 (2024)
63. Boven, R.V., Hamilton, R.H., Kauffman, T., Keenan, J.P., Pascual-Leone, A.: Neurology. **54**(12), 2230 (2000)
64. Remache-Vinueza, B., Trujillo-León, A., Vidal-Verdú, F.: Sci. Rep. **15**(1), 5057 (2025)
65. Alary, F., Duquette, M., Goldstein, R., Chapman, C.E., Voss, P., La Buissonnière-Ariza, V., Lepore, F.: Neuropsychologia. **47**(10), 2037 (2009)
66. Loomis, J.M.: Percept. Psychophys. **29**, 37 (1981)
67. Mutaguchi, K.: J. Spec. Educ. Res. **12**(2), 89 (2012)
68. McCarthy, T., Holbrook, C., Kamei-Hannan, C., D'Andrea, F.M.: J. Spec. Educ. Technol. **38**(4), 423 (2023)
69. Stanfa, K., Johnson, N.: J. Blind. Innov. Res. **5**, 2 (2015)
70. Knowlton, M., Wetzel, R.: J. Vis. Impair. Blind. **90**(3), 227 (1996)
71. Grunwald, A.P.: Science. **154**(3745), 144 (1966)
72. Ministry of Education, Culture, Sports, Science and Technology, Japan: Tenji Gakushu Shido No Tebiki (Guide to Braille Learning and Teaching). Nihon Bunkyou Shuppan. Osaka, Japan. (2003)
73. Bola, L., Siuda-Krzywicka, K., Papliński, M., Sumera, E., Hańczur, P., Szwed, M.: PLoS One. **11**(5), e0155394 (2016)
74. Kay, L.: Radio Electron. Eng. **44**(11), 605 (1974)
75. Pressey, N.: Focus. **11**(3), 35 (1977)
76. Ifukube, T., Sasaki, T., Peng, C.: IEEE Trans. Biomed. Eng. **38**(5), 461 (1991)

77. Dakopoulos, D., Bourbakis, N.G.: IEEE Trans. Syst. Man Cybern. Part C Appl. Rev. **40**(1), 25 (2009)
78. Meijer, P.B.: IEEE Trans. Biomed. Eng. **39**(2), 112 (1992)
79. Boldu, R., Dancu, A., Matthies, D.J., Buddhika, T., Siriwardhana, S., Nanayakkara, S.: Proc. ACM Interact. Mob. Wearable Ubiquitous Technol. **2**(3), 94:1 (2018)
80. Ulrich, I., Borenstein, J.: IEEE Trans. Syst. Man Cybern. A Syst. Humans. **31**(2), 131 (2001)
81. Manduchi, R., Coughlan, J.: Commun. ACM. **55**(1), 96 (2012)
82. Kugler, L.: Commun. ACM. **63**(12), 15 (2020)
83. Seki, Y., Sato, T.: IEEE Trans. Neural Syst. Rehabil. Eng. **19**(1), 95 (2010)
84. Seki, Y.: Universal Access in Human-Computer Interaction. Access to the Human Environment and Culture: 9th International Conference, UAHCI 2015, Held as Part of HCI International 2015, Los Angeles, CA, USA, August 2–7, 2015, Proceedings, Part IV 9, pp. 150–159. Springer (2015)
85. Honda, A., Shibata, H., Gyoba, J., Saitou, K., Iwaya, Y., Suzuki, Y.: Appl. Acoust. **68**(8), 885 (2007)
86. Wersényi, G.: J. Audio Eng. Soc. **60**(7/8), 568 (2012)
87. Miura, T., Suzuki, J., Muraoka, T., Ifukube, T.: ICAT, Dec (2010)
88. Mukhiddinov, M., Kim, S.Y.: PRO. **9**(10), 1726 (2021)
89. Watanabe, T., Yamaguchi, T., Koda, S., Minatani, K.: Computers Helping People with Special Needs: 14th International Conference, ICCHP 2014, Paris, France, July 9–11, 2014, Proceedings, Part II 14, pp. 42–49. Springer (2014)
90. Onishi, J., Sakai, T., Sakajiri, M., Ogata, A., Miura, T., Handa, T., Hiruma, N., Shimizu, T., Ono, T.: International Conference on Computers Helping People with Special Needs, pp. 92–99. Springer (2016)
91. Sakai, T., Handa, T., Sakajiri, M., Shimizu, T., Hiruma, N., Onishi, J.: J. Adv. Comput. Intell. Intell. Inform. **21**(1), 87 (2017)
92. Brandebusemeyer, C., Luther, A.R., König, S.U., König, P., Kärcher, S.M.: Sensors. **21**(21), 7384 (2021)
93. Jeong, G.Y., Yu, K.H.: Sensors. **16**(7), 1070 (2016)
94. Wersényi, G.: Sensors. **22**(22), 8962 (2022)
95. Watanabe, T., Watanabe, B., Fujinuma, T., Osugi, N., Sawada, M., Kamata, K.: J. IEICE, 891–899 (2005)
96. Asakawa, C., Itoh, T.: Proceedings of the Third International ACM Conference on Assistive Technologies, pp. 149–156 (1998)
97. Miyashita, H., Sato, D., Takagi, H., Asakawa, C.: Proceedings of the 2007 International Cross-Disciplinary Conference on Web Accessibility (W4A), pp. 126–127 (2007)
98. Borodin, Y., Bigham, J.P., Dausch, G., Ramakrishnan, I.: Proceedings of the 2010 International Cross Disciplinary Conference on Web Accessibility (W4A), p. 13:1–10 (2010)
99. Takagi, H., Saito, S., Fukuda, K., Asakawa, C.: ACM Trans. Comput.-Hum. Interact. **14**(3), 13 (2007)
100. Matsuo, M., Miura, T., Ichikari, R., Kato, K., Kurata, T.: J. Technol. Pers. Disabil., 82–103 (2020)
101. Kane, S.K., Bigham, J.P., Wobbrock, J.O.: Proceedings of the 10th International ACM SIGAC- CESS Conference on Computers and Accessibility, pp. 73–80 (2008)
102. Blindsquare. https://www.blindsquare.com/
103. Ahmetovic, D., Gleason, C., Ruan, C., Kitani, K., Takagi, H., Asakawa, C.: Proceedings of the 18th International Conference on Human-Computer Interaction with Mobile Devices and Services, pp. 90–99 (2016)
104. Sato, D., Oh, U., Naito, K., Takagi, H., Kitani, K., Asakawa, C.: Proceedings of the 19th International ACM SIGACCESS Conference on Computers and Accessibility, pp. 270–279 (2017)
105. Erdenesambuu, D., Matsuo, M., Miura, T., Sakajiri, M., Onishi, J.: International Conference on Computers Helping People with Special Needs, pp. 416–427. Springer (2024)

106. Guerreiro, J., Sato, D., Asakawa, S., Dong, H., Kitani, K.M., Asakawa, C.: Proceedings of the 21st International ACM SIGACCESS Conference on Computers and Accessibility, pp. 68–82 (2019)
107. Shoval, S., Ulrich, I., Borenstein, J.: IEEE Robot. Autom. Mag. **10**(1), 9 (2003)
108. Kayukawa, S., Sato, D., Murata, M., Ishihara, T., Takagi, H., Morishima, S., Asakawa, C.: Proceedings of the 2023 CHI Conference on Human Factors in Computing Systems, pp. 1–14 (2023)
109. Bigham, J.P., Jayant, C., Ji, H., Little, G., Miller, A., Miller, R.C., Miller, R., Tatarowicz, A., White, B., White, S., et al.: Proceedings of the 23nd Annual ACM Symposium on User Interface Software and Technology, pp. 333–342 (2010)
110. Holton, B.: AFB AccessWorld Magazine. **14** (2013)
111. Gurari, D., Li, Q., Stangl, A.J., Guo, A., Lin, C., Grauman, K., Luo, J., Bigham, J.P.: Proceedings of the IEEE Conference on Computer Vision and Pattern Recognition, pp. 3608–3617 (2018)
112. Seeing AI App from Microsoft. https://www.microsoft.com/en-us/ai/seeing-ai
113. Envision - perceive possibility. https://www.letsenvision.com/
114. Sadjo, E., Findlater, L., Stangl, A.: Proceedings of the 23rd International ACM SIGACCESS Conference on Computers and Accessibility, pp. 1–4 (2021)

Chapter 5
Supporting Physical Activity in the Elderly and Persons with Disabilities

Yusuke Maeda and Toshiaki Tanaka

Abstract Section 5.1 describes ergonomic approaches aimed at preventing falls and improving balance ability. Conventionally, center of pressure (COP) analysis using a force platform has long been used to evaluate postural control ability. However, it has been shown that COP parameters during static standing balance are not strongly associated with fall risk. Therefore, dynamic elements such as COP during perturbed standing or sensory disturbances have been incorporated to assess fall risk. Additionally, new insights have been gained by analyzing postural sway using frequency analysis. Furthermore, this section will introduce fall-related research using small accelerometers, insights into mHealth, and the benefits of balance training utilizing video games and external disturbances.

The authors have primarily conducted research on evaluating dynamic postural control for fall prevention and assessing the effectiveness of related training. Their work has mainly involved comparing younger and older individuals to investigate age-related changes in postural control, with a particular focus on the impact of aging on responses to visual and plantar somatosensory perturbations. They have also built extensive evidence regarding postural control in response to external disturbances, as well as foot trajectory and stepping velocity during stepping movements. In their research on training effectiveness, they have developed a simple and safe stepping exercise method that community-dwelling older adults can perform at home, with future practical application anticipated.

Section 5.3 provides a comprehensive review of studies investigating the use of sensory stimulation interventions to improve balance in the elderly. Several experiments measured foot tactile thresholds, dynamic postural sway, and limits of stability to evaluate the effects of vibratory stimulation to the feet and trunk. The

Y. Maeda
School of Health Sciences at Odawara, International University of Health and Welfare, Kanagawa, Japan
e-mail: y.maeda@ihwg.jp

T. Tanaka (✉)
Research Center for Advanced Science and Technology/Institute of Gerontology, The University of Tokyo, Tokyo, Japan
e-mail: t.tanaka@iog.u-tokyo.ac.jp; tanaka@bfp.rcast.u-tokyo.ac.jp

T. Tanaka (ed.), *Inclusive and Barrier-Free Designs for Rehabilitation Engineering*,
https://doi.org/10.1007/978-981-95-5783-7_5

findings demonstrated that short-term and long-term sensory interventions significantly enhanced sensory feedback and balance performance. Additionally, the chapter discusses studies that used virtual reality to provide moving auditory and tactile inputs. These studies highlight the potential of virtual reality to support posture control and gait training in daily life. The results suggest that combining vibratory stimulation with VR-based multisensory feedback is an innovative approach to fall prevention and rehabilitation. Future research should focus on optimizing stimulation parameters, enabling home-based training, and conducting large-scale randomized controlled trials to validate the efficacy of these interventions and develop personalized programs for elderly individuals.

5.1 A Review of Assistive Engineering Research on Standing Balance

5.1.1 Introduction

Falls in older adults can lead to serious consequences, including fractures and a bedridden state. As individuals age, their postural control function declines, thereby increasing their fall risk. "Postural control" refers to the ability to maintain the body's center of gravity (COG) within a specific range. If the COG deviates from this range, a fall occurs, necessitating the establishment of a new support base. To achieve this, perceiving one's own COG position and the status of each body part through sensory input (input system) from various sensory organs, such as the visual, somatosensory, and vestibular systems, is crucial. The central nervous system, including the cerebrum and cerebellum, integrates sensory information (the integration system) and outputs the necessary motor commands to each muscle (the output system). Approaches to fall prevention require improvement in the aforementioned postural control ability, and balance and strength training is considered effective. In recent years, the importance of ergonomic approaches using various devices has increased.

5.1.2 COP Sway Measurement [1]

Traditionally, quiet standing control is evaluated by measuring the trajectory of the COP. The parameters for evaluating quiet standing control ability include COP displacement, velocity, area, and frequency characteristics. Prieto et al. [2] introduced various measures of postural stability based on the planar trajectory of COP during standing tasks. They demonstrated that various aspects of quiet standing could be evaluated using not only the COP trajectory length but also the area values with the root mean square distance, average velocity, and average frequency. Colins et al. researched the mechanisms of quiet standing in humans and proposed a novel concept that considers the maintenance of an upright posture as a stochastic process. This research posited that two types of control mechanisms are at play—namely, short term (0–0.5 s) and long term (2–10 s). This suggests that short-term control involves open-loop control (a direct reaction to the input), whereas long-term control involves closed-loop control (adjustments using neural feedback) [3]. Using the same methodology, they investigated the influence of visual input on maintaining a standing posture [4]. Their findings indicate that increased visual input can reduce the contribution of the musculoskeletal, proprioceptive, and vestibular systems. Rocchi et al. aimed to avoid redundancy and simplify the interpretation of results when evaluating postural stability using the COP. The assessment was subdivided into four aspects [5]: ① measures of trajectory length, such as root mean square distance, ② frequency dispersion, ③ directional specificity of the COP trajectory in the mediolateral and anteroposterior directions, and ④ frequency components.

① It has been demonstrated to be sensitive to various treatments for Parkinson's disease (PD), such as levodopa and deep brain stimulation [6]. It has also been used to detect postural abnormalities in patients with peripheral neuropathy [7].
② A unitless measure of the frequency dispersion, estimated by FD, a parameter related to the shape of the PSD curve that quantifies the degree of determinism in the COP displacements. Relevant frequencies that characterize the power spectral density curve: f50, f95, and centroidal frequency.
③The mean velocity in the anteroposterior (AP) direction correlates with clinical scores that characterize patients with stroke [2, 8].
④ Specifically responds to aging [8].

A clear definition of COP-based assessment has enabled the modeling of quiet standing, thereby accelerating research on postural control [1].

5.1.3 Balance Assessment Using Wearable Inertial Measurement Units (IMUs)

Since the early 2000s, many studies have used IMUs, particularly accelerometers, for balance assessment. Hansson et al. confirmed the high reliability of IMUs by demonstrating a strong correlation between the data from an IMU worn on the lower back and a force plate [9]. Noamani et al. validated the accuracy of IMUs and demonstrated their high precision compared to acceleration data obtained from analysis devices, such as cameras and force plates [10]. Many of these systems involve attaching a sensor to the lumbar region (sacrum) and can be used to evaluate postural control strategies [1]. Common parameters include acceleration-related measures such as the RMS of acceleration, jerk (the derivative of acceleration), and centroidal frequency. The reliability of the iPad IMU was also confirmed in a previous study [11]. Combining the assessment of the forces acting on the COG and COP can yield significant insights. Various studies have been conducted using IMUs on patients with diabetes. The maximum shear and vertical pressures applied to the foot during walking are directly related to the onset and progression of ulcers (skin breakdown), making the methods for evaluating the characteristics of these phases particularly beneficial for patients with diabetic foot syndrome. Washabaugh et al. evaluated the reliability of IMUs worn on the foot or ankle when measuring spatiotemporal gait parameters such as walking speed, step length, and cadence [12]. Felius et al. assessed the reliability of IMUs when measuring trunk balance parameters in a static standing position [13].

5.1.4 Mobile Health (mHealth)

mHealth refers to medical and health services that utilize mobile devices such as smartphones and tablets. This offers benefits such as facilitating easy health management and enabling residents in remote areas to receive appropriate medical and nursing care services. Specific examples include the monitoring of vital signs [14], detection of symptoms and anomalies [15, 16], and patient education [17]. mHealth training can be categorized into applications specifically for gait training, balance training, and physical activity programs performed at home. Examples used in gait training include metronome applications that provide rhythmic auditory stimulation [18] and applications that offer visually engaging feedback from world-famous scenery [19]. Trunk training applications utilize visual feedback [20] and are designed for seated balance training [21]. These tools enable individuals to perform guided home-based programs, monitor their behaviors and symptoms, and facilitate communication with therapists. A meta-analysis conducted by Moreno-Ligero et al. [22] showed that mHealth may positively affect gait and balance in patients with neurological disorders. Supervising adherence to physical activity through mHealth apps has been reported to result in improved walking ability in patients with chronic stroke who participated in an 8-week rehabilitation program, including aerobic, task oriented, balance, and stretching exercises, compared with the control group [23]. Emerging evidence suggests that exercise interventions delivered through apps and websites, also known as digital approaches, are effective in improving physical activity levels in older adults. According to McGarrigle et al. [24], several websites and smartphone applications for fall prevention have been evaluated. The average score for 24 websites ultimately rated in their review was 71.74%, indicating good quality. Eight websites were rated as excellent, 12 as good, and 4 as adequate, with no websites rated as poor. Furthermore, out of seven apps that included evidence-based exercises for fall prevention, four were rated as "good" on the Mobile Application Rating Scale for quality assessment. These four apps (StandingTall, Otago Exercise Program, Nymbl Balance, and Keep On Keep Up) also achieved relatively good scores regarding the use of behavior change techniques. The main advantage of Web-based videos and images is that they are freely accessible to anyone with access to an Internet-connected computer without requiring a smartphone or tablet. With the accumulation of evidence regarding exercise for fall prevention, there is concern that the benefits will be lost quickly if exercise is stopped; therefore, the challenge is how to ensure continued exercise. A recent Green Paper on Prevention from Public Health England (PHE) proposed prioritizing digital approaches to support the public in regularly engaging in strength and balance exercises. The European Network for Fall Prevention (Pro-FaNE) brings together scientists, clinicians, and other healthcare professionals from across Europe to conduct workshops focused on key themes such as the clinical assessment and management of falls, evaluation of balance function, and psychological aspects of falls to exchange knowledge, expertise, and resources regarding interventions to reduce falls [25]. These examples illustrate how fall prevention approaches are being advanced at national and global levels through digital tools and network environments.

5.1.5 Video Game-Based Balance Training

Regarding video game-based balance training, the popularity of active video games (AVGs) that require physical movement is increasing, and reports [26] suggest their potential positive effects on overall health and various disabilities (such as cerebral palsy, multiple sclerosis, and PD). The unique interactive features of AVGs allow players to experience both training and enjoyment, enabling them to continue training without consciously focusing on physical exertion [27]. Furthermore, they facilitated the continuation of exercise even during the isolation periods enforced by the COVID-19 pandemic [28]. Wu et al. conducted a meta-analysis of 11 studies on children with cerebral palsy and reported positive effects of AVGs on balance improvement [29]. Taylor et al. performed a meta-analysis of ten studies on older adults and demonstrated that AVGs improved indicators of mobility and balance [30]. Hocking et al. focused on the effects of AVGs in children with developmental disabilities (such as spastic and hemiplegic cerebral palsy) and showed a small-to-medium effect on balance abilities [31].

Exergames are a form of game-based exercises for community-dwelling older adults that involves the use of commercially available video games and virtual reality (VR). In addition to improving balance, exergames have been reported to enhance sensory integration skills, improve fall efficacy, and positively affect cognitive aspects such as mood and attention [32].

5.1.6 Step-Inducing Training for Fall Prevention Using a Perturbation-Based System

In unpredictable situations in which balance may be lost, recovering balance through appropriate stepping movements is crucial for fall avoidance. The experimental methods for creating such unexpected situations include the slip method, trip method, surface translation, and waist pull. Studies using the slip method created unexpected slips and analyzed recovery movements to examine the potential and severity of falls [33]. An analysis using motion capture and force plates showed that feet-forward slips (where the slipping and landing legs are on the same side) are significantly more dangerous than split slips (where the slipping and remaining legs are on opposite sides) because they result in a greater estimated impact on the hip joint and a larger backward trunk angle. In the trip method, Pijnappels et al. measured the reactions of young and older adults when they unexpectedly encountered an obstacle during walking and tripped [34]. Elderly fallers exhibit decreased joint moment during push-off, inappropriate placement of the recovery limb (the leg that contacts the ground), and a delay in knee joint moment generation, leading to the argument that lower limb strength training can help in reducing the fall risk. Furthermore, a report on the effectiveness of fall prevention training combining trips and slips indicated that when 44 community-dwelling older adults underwent a total of 120 min of training sessions that combined trip and slip perturbations, the training group experienced a 60% reduction in perturbation-induced falls (30% body weight load on a harness) compared with the control group that underwent traditional training [35]. Regarding fall risk assessment using surface translation, Batcir et al. kinematically analyzed step movements using a video camera when an unexpected lateral (side-to-side) translation perturbation was applied to the floor and compared single- and multiple-step responses [36]. In the case of a single step, the step time increased as the perturbation magnitude increased, leading to the interpretation that the initial step involved selecting a stepping motion appropriate for the perturbation size. However, when a larger perturbation required multiple steps, there was no increase in step time with increasing perturbation size, leading to the argument that multiple steps involved a rigid and automatic response. To examine stepping movements due to waist-pull perturbation, Mille et al. compared the stepping strategies of young and older adults [37]. In response to lateral perturbations, older adults tended to use a crossover step, which was characterized by a longer step time, delayed initiation, a higher step, and a similar increase in lateral trunk displacement as in younger adults. It was found that older adults are compelled to adopt a high-risk strategy for lower limb collisions owing to the crossover step.

5.2 Basic and Clinical Research on Fall Prevention Training Focusing on Sensory Function

5.2.1 Introduction

The number of severe injuries, such as femoral neck fractures, due to falls and slips among the elderly is increasing annually, often leading to a bedridden state or restricted range of activities and causing a significant decline in activities of daily living (ADLs) and quality of life (QOL). Furthermore, associated medical and nursing care costs are substantial, resulting in significant economic losses. Therefore, fall prevention in the elderly is critically important. To develop effective fall prevention approaches for the elderly, it is essential to understand the postural control mechanisms in healthy individuals and identify age-related changes in these abilities. The following section outlines several research directions aimed at developing fall prevention strategies.

In Sect. 5.2.2 of this chapter, significant insights into the fall risk of independent elderly individuals using posturography described in Sect. 5.1.2 are presented. Although it offers the advantage of easy quantification of static postural control ability, the correlation between static postural control ability and fall risk in the elderly is relatively small. Falls in elderly individuals were successfully detected by conducting posturography using the limit of stability (LOS) test, which incorporates dynamic elements. We conclude that dynamic postural control is necessary for assessing the fall risk. In Sect. 2.3 of this chapter, posturography incorporating some dynamic elements was conducted, and fundamental data regarding the foot arch, which is an important factor in maintaining the standing posture, were obtained. In Sects. 2.4 and 2.5 of this chapter, regarding dynamic postural control, which is strongly associated with falls, responses to unpredictable floor perturbation stimuli were investigated, and important insights into postural adjustments under restricted sensory input were gained. Sections 5.2.6 and 5.2.7 discussed the analysis of stepping performance and the effects of step training in older adults.

5.2.2 Fall Risk in the Elderly Population [38]

COP measurements and physical function data were collected to comprehensively evaluate the balance ability of elderly individuals and assess their fall risk. Furthermore, the influence of various parameters on the frequency of falls was examined using discriminant analysis. The participants comprised 79 elderly individuals (age: 73.2 ± 4.2 years) without severe diseases who were living independently at home and 70 healthy young adults (age: 20.7 ± 1.4 years). COP measurements, two-point discrimination of plantar sensation, grip strength, lower limb range of motion (ROM), and a clinical balance test (Berg balance test) were conducted. The following relationship was obtained: Z (discriminant function) = 0.002 × total score of the LOS test +0.139 × grip strength − 4.15. Furthermore, the female group exhibited a significantly higher fall rate and higher COP velocity than the male group. In conclusion, the total score of the LOS test and grip strength was associated with the frequency of falls, suggesting that these parameters may be useful in fall screening.

5.2.3 *Effect of Load Change on Foot Arch in Different Positions [39]*

This study analyzed the effect of load changes in different foot positions on the foot arch using clinical assessments with a Vicon motion analysis system, goniometer, and calipers in healthy young adults. The reliability of the measurements was evaluated using the Vicon motion analysis system and clinical assessments. Two methods were used to measure the foot arch: (1) Vicon motion analysis and (2) goniometer and calipers. Measurements were taken bilaterally in six different postures: standing on both feet, standing on one foot, heel raising, medial weight shifting, lateral weight shifting, and ankle dorsiflexion. The heights of the medial longitudinal, lateral longitudinal, and transverse arches in the dynamic posture were significantly greater than those in static standing. The results from the Vicon motion analysis system showed a high correlation with the measurements obtained by clinical assessment only for static postures. When the foot and ankle joints were in a dynamic and unstable position, the windlass mechanism caused the arches to be higher than those in a static position. Effective assessment required simultaneous evaluation of the three foot arches in various positions.

5.2.4 *Postural Control Against External Disturbances in the Presence of Sensory Perturbation [40]*

Although numerous reports exist regarding the role of the sensory system in postural control, only a few have reported the relationship between sensory perturbation and dynamic postural control. To investigate dynamic postural control ability, postural responses to translational platform perturbations were quantitatively evaluated. Eight healthy young adults (males aged 21.3 $\pm$ 1.4 years) were subjected to experimental floor translation perturbations using a platform that could move in four directions (anterior, posterior, right, left). A stabilometer was used to measure COP trajectories and electromyography (EMG) of the trunk and lower limb muscles, and video analysis was conducted to measure joint angles (Fig. 5.1). To assess the effects of sensory perturbation, conditions were established with participants wearing translucent goggles and standing on a compliant mat. A significant difference in COP displacement was observed between conditions with and without sensory perturbation. With sensory perturbation, the mediolateral and anteroposterior components of displacement increased during posterior and lateral translations, respectively. Furthermore, postural responses to anterior translation were not affected by sensory perturbation, as compared to those to posterior and mediolateral translations. These analytical results provide useful insights into the development of dynamic balance rehabilitation under sensory perturbation conditions.

Fig. 5.1 Platform

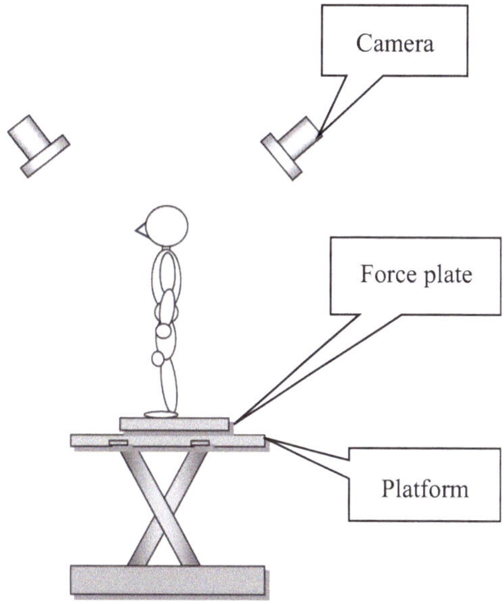

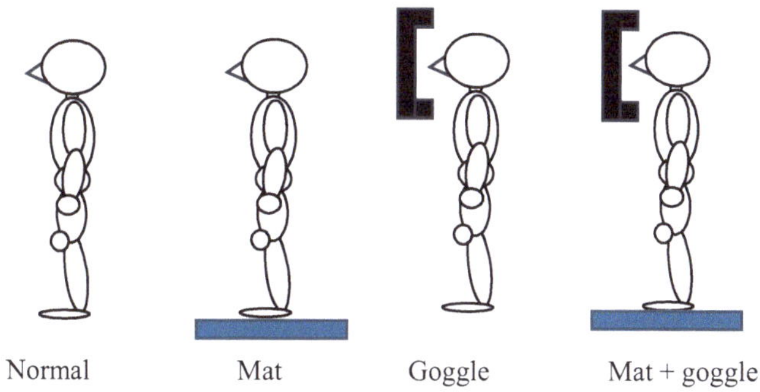

Fig. 5.2 Sensory perturbation

5.2.5 Age-Related Changes in Dynamic Postural Control Ability in the Presence of Sensory Perturbation [41]

To develop fall prevention programs, it is necessary to carefully examine dynamic postural control in elderly individuals under sensory perturbation conditions. This study investigated how elderly individuals respond to external perturbations when their vision and somatosensation are disturbed (Fig. 5.2). The participants included four healthy elderly individuals and six young adults. Perturbation stimuli were applied via a platform that could move in four directions (anterior, posterior, right, and left). The effects of the sensory perturbations induced by wearing translucent goggles and standing on compliant surfaces were examined. The measured parameters included COP trajectories on a force plate, lower limb EMG, and joint angles obtained through video analysis. COP analysis revealed that the elderly group took a longer time (recovery time) to return to an upright posture after external perturbations, particularly when the sensory input was disrupted. EMG analysis indicated that the elderly group utilized the knee joint muscles to respond to postural perturbations involving vertical movement. Recovery time is a characteristic parameter of the response to external perturbations under sensory perturbation conditions and is a potentially useful indicator for evaluating balance ability. The increased activity of the muscles around the knee joint is likely due to a reduction in ankle plantar flexion/dorsiflexion torque, which is considered one of the reasons for the prolonged recovery time. These findings can be applied to the development of fall prevention training programs.

5.2.6 *Different Effects of 12-Week Speed or Accuracy Training on Obstacle Crossing [42]*

Tripping is a common cause of falls, making it important to improve the stepping movements. This study aimed to compare speed- and accuracy-focused sideway stepping training to establish effective training methods. A randomized controlled trial (RCT) was conducted to investigate the effects of the stepping training. Twenty healthy older adults (71.7 ± 1.5 years old) were randomly assigned to either a speed training group or an accuracy training group. Over a period of 12 weeks, each group practiced sideways stepping movements either as fast or as accurately as possible (aiming for the same movement each time). A three-dimensional motion capture system was used to record stepping movement data before and after the training period. To analyze stepping movements, four conditions were established: stepping from a normal standing position, fast stepping from a normal standing position, stepping from an inclined standing position, and fast stepping from an inclined standing position. These conditions were tested in two directions: forward and sideways. Stepping movements in the speed training group were significantly faster than those at baseline. However, stepping movement accuracy in the accuracy training group did not show statistically significant improvement. It is a useful finding that stepping training from a normal upright posture also improves swing speed from an inclined posture. This training is easy and practical for older adults.

5.2.7 *Age-Related Changes in Accuracy and Speed of Lateral Crossing Motion [43]*

This study analyzed the accuracy and speed of movement in elderly individuals while stepping over a lateral obstacle from a tilted standing posture. Twenty healthy older adults (6 males, 14 females, aged 71.7 ± 1.5 years) and 20 healthy young adults (5 males, 15 females, aged 21.4 ± 1.2 years) participated in this research. Four conditions were established as follows: stepping from a normal standing position, fast stepping from a normal standing position, stepping from a tilted standing position, and fast stepping from a tilted standing position. Participants performed a total of ten lateral obstacle-crossing steps in each condition. The participants were instructed to perform each stepping motion ten times while maintaining as consistent a movement as possible. The stepping movements were captured using a three-dimensional analysis system. The trajectories of the swing foot, landing position, stepping time, body COM, and lower limb moments were calculated and compared between young and elderly adults. In the stepping motion from a tilted standing position, the stepping time and knee joint moment of elderly adults were significantly longer and larger than those of young adults. Under the same conditions, the results for foot trajectory and landing position revealed inconsistencies in the foot movements of the elderly adults. Aging makes it difficult for older individuals to perform the intended stepping and rapid swing movements. This movement inconsistency is thought to be a significant cause of falls among elderly individuals.

5.3 A Comprehensive Study on Improving Balance in the Elderly Through Plantar and Trunk Sensory Stimulation

5.3.1 Background

As society ages, falls have become a serious problem for the elderly. In Japan, fractures and bruises resulting from falls are among the leading causes of long-term care requirements [44–46]. As people age, their sensitivity to tactile and vibratory sensations in their soles and toes decreases. This decrease adversely affects their postural control while standing and walking. Sensory input from the soles is important because it integrates with visual and vestibular information to maintain balance. Sensory decline makes it difficult to perceive body tilt or movement direction, thereby increasing the risk of falls. Recently, interventions that use sensory stimulation to improve feedback have gained attention. These efforts have focused on vibration-based research [47, 48]. This chapter introduces new balance training methods that use sensory stimulation for rehabilitating standing in elderly individuals and discusses the development of health and welfare devices. It also covers future perspectives in barrier-free and inclusive design for mobility support.

5.3.2 Objective

This study aims to summarize the findings of vibration studies [44, 49–52] and evaluate the effectiveness of sensory stimulation interventions in maintaining and improving standing balance ability in rehabilitation. Specifically, we examine how sensory stimulation applied to the soles and trunk contributes to improvements in sensory thresholds and static/dynamic balance ability in the elderly from the perspectives of rehabilitation and welfare engineering. The study also aims to clarify the potential for clinical applications and future research issues.

5.3.3 Methods

In the Vibration Study [44], sensory thresholds of the toes and soles were measured in young and elderly adults (20 subjects per group), and center-of-gravity sway while standing was compared. In the Vibration Study [49], we evaluated the effect of weak, short-duration vibratory sensory feedback applied to the soles on standing balance (Fig. 5.3). In the Vibration Study [50], an eight-week balance training program using a force plate and a vibration stimulation device was conducted with

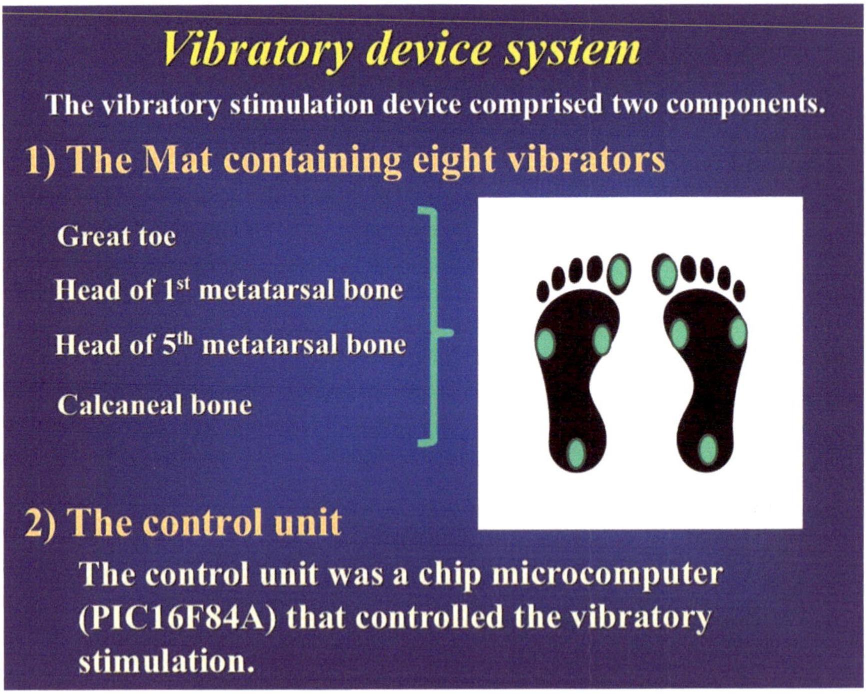

Fig. 5.3 Vibratory sensory feedback device. (Modified from Tanaka et al. [49])

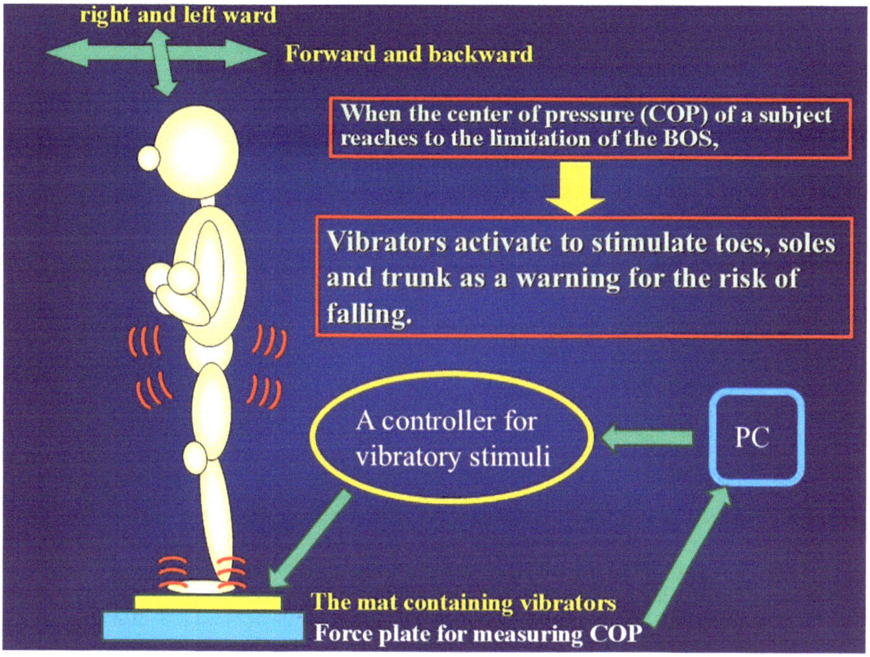

Fig. 5.4 Balance training device combining vibrators and center-of-gravity measurement system. (Modified from Tanaka et al. [49])

60 elderly individuals. The program measured the maximum range of anterior-posterior and mediolateral sway to evaluate dynamic balance ability (Fig. 5.4). In the Vibration Study [51], 18 participants were divided into plantar, trunk, and control groups. The effects of 10-week sensory training interventions to the soles and trunk were evaluated before and after the intervention using the limits of stability (LoS) test and two-point discrimination ability (Figs. 5.5 and 5.6).

5.3.4 Results

In the Vibration Study [44], the elderly group exhibited significantly higher sensory thresholds in the soles compared to the younger group and demonstrated greater postural sway under visual occlusion (Fig. 5.7). In the Vibration Study [49], weak vibratory stimulation applied to the soles improved sensory feedback while standing and reduced sway. In the Vibration Study [50], post-training results showed a significant increase in maximum anterior-posterior and mediolateral sway ranges, indicating improved dynamic balance. In the Vibration Study [51], significant improvements in LoS test scores and two-point discrimination ability were observed in the trunk and sole intervention groups.

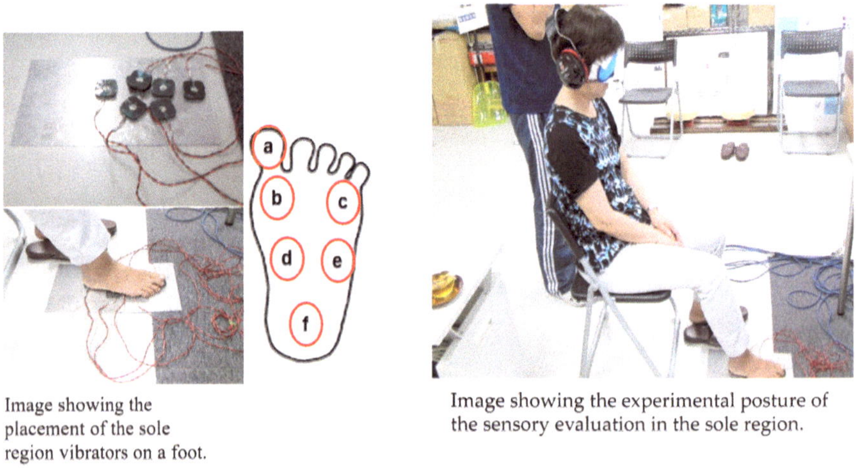

Fig. 5.5 Overview of the vibrator arrangement and vibration stimulation pattern for plantar vibration sensation evaluation. Vibrators labeled a–f are placed on key points of the foot. The central images display the vibrator arrangement, while the right image shows the participant seated, blindfolded, and wearing headphones during the evaluation

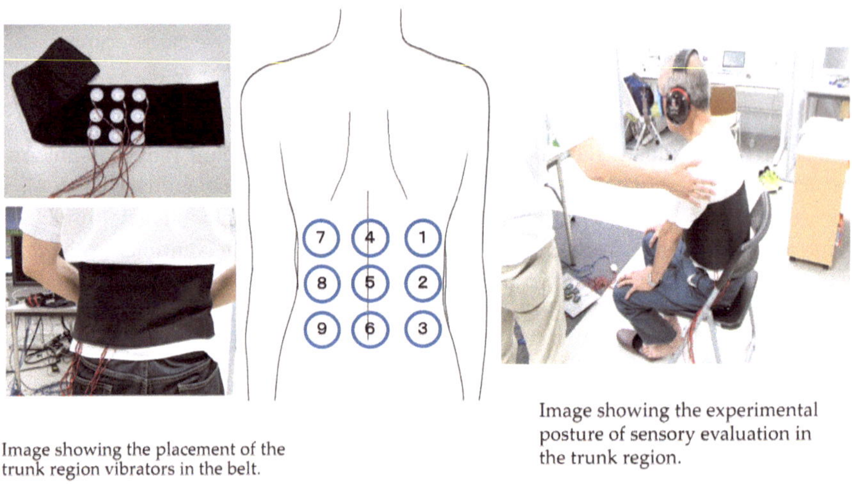

Fig. 5.6 Overview of the vibrator arrangement and vibration stimulation pattern for trunk vibration sensation evaluation. Nine vibrators are arranged in a 3 × 3 grid on a belt. The left images show the belt and its placement; the right shows a participant wearing the belt with headphones and blindfolds to block external stimuli

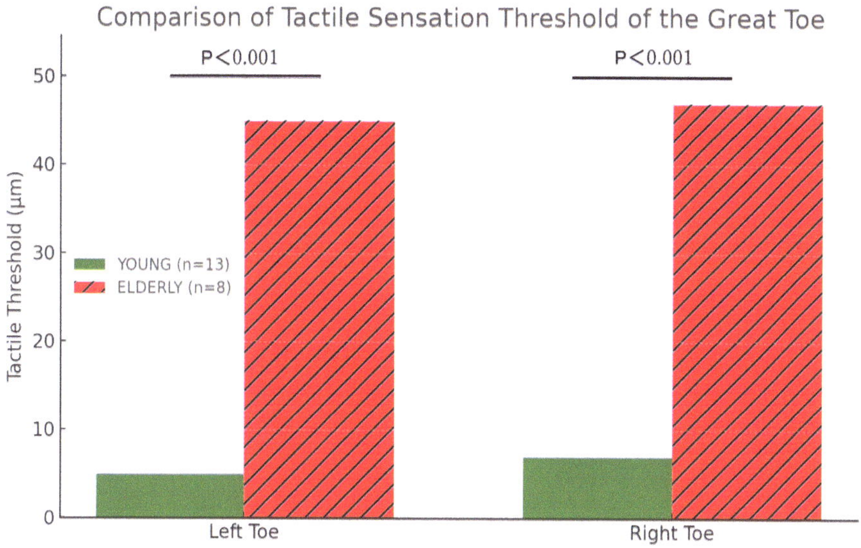

Fig. 5.7 Comparison of tactile thresholds between young and elderly participants (left and right great toe)

5.3.5 *Discussion*

This study demonstrated that sensory stimulation interventions effectively improve sensory function and balance in the elderly. These results align with those of previous studies [47, 48]). Interventions that involve not only the soles but also the trunk may promote sensory integration in the central nervous system, thereby enhancing full-body postural control. Recent research also suggests that long-term sensory stimulation interventions may positively impact muscle strength and gait. Future research should focus on optimizing intervention periods, enabling in-home practice, and designing personalized programs. Adjusting stimulation thresholds and frequencies may maximize intervention effectiveness. Large-scale randomized controlled trials (RCTs) and multisite collaborative studies are expected to shape future directions.

Additionally, we present research that highlights the role of sensory input in maintaining balance, the use of virtual reality (VR) to supplement sensory function, and the medical potential of VR.

One study examined the effect of moving auditory stimuli on standing balance in young and elderly adults [52]. Twelve healthy individuals (seven young and five elderly participants) were exposed to white noise presented via a 3D audio virtual reality (VR) system in which the sound image moved lateral direction rather than anteroposterior direction (Fig. 5.8). Their balance was measured using a center-of-pressure (COP) device and plantar pressure sensors while standing on stable and unstable surfaces with their eyes open and closed. The results showed that, under

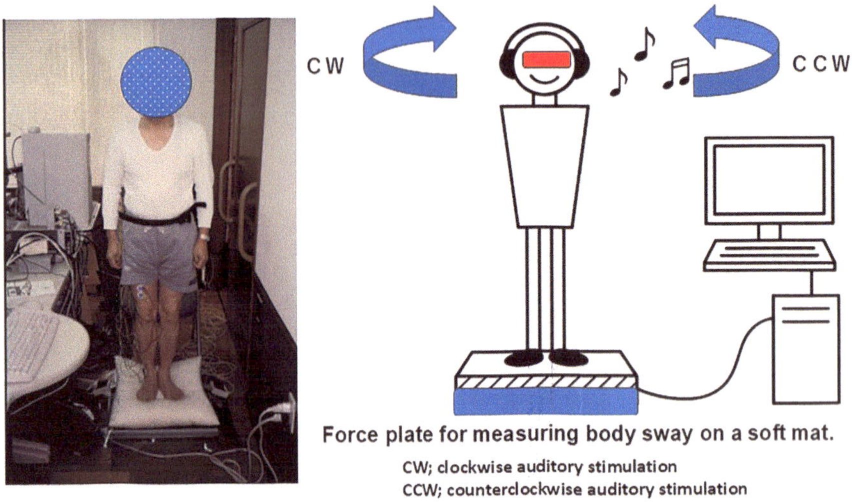

Fig. 5.8 The standing balance experiment uses virtual reality (VR) with auditory stimulation

Table 5.1 Moving vibratory stimuli in six patterns

Pattern	Description
Rightward	Left head of 5th metatarsal bone → Left head of 1st metatarsal bone → Right head of 1st metatarsal bone → Right head of 5th metatarsal bone
Leftward	Reverse of the right side pattern
Forward	Both calcaneal bones → Both head of 1st metatarsal bone → Both great toes
Backward	Reverse of the forward pattern
Clockwise	Left calcaneal bone → Left head of 5th metatarsal bone → Left great toe → Right great toe → Right head of 5th metatarsal bone → Right calcaneal bone
Counter clockwise	Reverse of the clockwise pattern

Modified from Tanaka et al. [50]

visual deprivation and reduced tactile input, the elderly participants exhibited significantly greater mediolateral sway in response to the moving sound. They also relied more on their heels than their toes, indicating a different postural strategy than that of younger adults. These results suggest that auditory and tactile feedback could be beneficial for balance training in the elderly.

Another study investigated the impact of brief, moving vibratory stimuli applied to the feet on postural control [49]. Young adults (mean age: 23.7) and elderly adults (mean age: 81.1) received 1-s stimuli via eight small vibrators on the soles in six directions: anterior, posterior, left, right, clockwise, and counterclockwise (Table 5.1). Postural sway was recorded in the anteroposterior and mediolateral directions using a COP device. Though there were no significant differences between stimulated and non-stimulated conditions, elderly participants showed greater sway overall. Young adults tended to shift their COP in the opposite direction of the vibration, while the elderly did not. Instead, the elderly appeared to adjust their posture to reduce pressure on the stimulated area, possibly due to altered sensation. These results suggest that reduced plantar sensation affects the elderly's perception of vibration and balance. Adjusting vibration intensity and direction could enhance plantar feedback and support balance training and fall prevention.

These studies indicate that VR-based modulation of auditory, tactile, and visual inputs could assist people with ADLs to become independent.

5.3.6 Conclusion

Interventions involving vibratory stimulation to the soles and trunk were found to effectively improve sensory and balance functions in the elderly. These results highlight the potential of sensory stimulation as an innovative fall prevention strategy and could lead to its clinical application in rehabilitation. Additionally, integrating VR-based modulation of auditory, tactile, and visual inputs shows promise in improving posture and gait training in daily life. This has valuable implications for the future development of rehabilitation and assistive technologies.

References

1. Noamani, A., et al.: Clinical static balance assessment: a narrative review of traditional and IMU-based posturography in older adults and individuals with incomplete spinal cord injury. Sensors (Basel). **23**(21) (2023)
2. Prieto, T.E., et al.: Measures of postural steadiness: differences between healthy young and elderly adults. I.E.E.E. Trans. Biomed. Eng. **43**(9), 956–966 (1996)
3. Collins, J.J., De Luca, C.J.: Open-loop and closed-loop control of posture: a random-walk analysis of center-of-pressure trajectories. Exp. Brain Res. **95**(2), 308–318 (1993)
4. Collins, J.J., De Luca, C.J.: The effects of visual input on open-loop and closed-loop postural control mechanisms. Exp. Brain Res. **103**(1), 151–163 (1995)
5. Rocchi, L., Chiari, L., Cappello, A.: Feature selection of stabilometric parameters based on principal component analysis. Med. Biol. Eng. Comput. **42**(1), 71–79 (2004)
6. Rocchi, L., Chiari, L., Horak, F.: Effects of deep brain stimulation and levodopa on postural sway in Parkinson's disease. J. Neurol. Neurosurg. Psychiatry. **73**(3), 267–274 (2002)
7. Yamamoto, R., et al.: Postural sway and diabetic peripheral neuropathy. Diabetes Res. Clin. Pract. **52**(3), 213–221 (2001)
8. Maki, B.E., Holliday, P.J., Topper, A.K.: A prospective study of postural balance and risk of falling in an ambulatory and independent elderly population. J. Gerontol. **49**(2), M72–M84 (1994)
9. Ekvall Hansson, E., Tornberg, Å.: Coherence and reliability of a wearable inertial measurement unit for measuring postural sway. BMC. Res. Notes. **12**(1), 201 (2019)
10. Noamani, A., et al.: Validity of using wearable inertial sensors for assessing the dynamics of standing balance. Med. Eng. Phys. **77**, 53–59 (2020)
11. Alberts, J.L., et al.: Using accelerometer and gyroscopic measures to quantify postural stability. J. Athl. Train. **50**(6), 578–588 (2015)

12. Washabaugh, E.P., et al.: Validity and repeatability of inertial measurement units for measuring gait parameters. Gait Posture. **55**, 87–93 (2017)
13. Felius, R.A.W., et al.: Reliability of IMU-based balance assessment in clinical stroke rehabilitation. Gait Posture. **98**, 62–68 (2022)
14. Andrew, B.Y., et al.: mStroke: "Mobile stroke"—improving acute stroke care with smartphone technology. J. Stroke Cerebrovasc. Dis. **26**(7), 1449–1456 (2017)
15. Banky, M., et al.: Toward accurate clinical spasticity assessment: validation of movement speed and joint angle assessments using smartphones and camera tracking. Arch. Phys. Med. Rehabil. **100**(8), 1482–1491 (2019)
16. Sarfo, F.S., et al.: Phone-based intervention for blood pressure control among Ghanaian stroke survivors: a pilot randomized controlled trial. Int. J. Stroke. **14**(6), 630–638 (2019)
17. Dorsey, E.R., et al.: Teleneurology and mobile technologies: the future of neurological care. Nat. Rev. Neurol. **14**(5), 285–297 (2018)
18. Hankinson, K., et al.: A tailored music-motor therapy and real-time biofeedback mobile phone app ('GotRhythm') to promote rehabilitation following stroke: a pilot study. Neurosci. Insights. **17**, 26331055221100587 (2022)
19. Lee, J., Lee, K., Song, C.: Speed-interactive treadmill training using smartphone-based motion tracking technology improves gait in stroke patients. J. Mot. Behav. **49**(6), 675–685 (2017)
20. Shin, D.C., Song, C.H.: Smartphone-based visual feedback trunk control training using a gyroscope and mirroring technology for stroke patients: single-blinded, randomized clinical trial of efficacy and feasibility. Am. J. Phys. Med. Rehabil. **95**(5), 319–329 (2016)
21. Aphiphaksakul, P., Siriphorn, A.: Home-based exercise using balance disc and smartphone inclinometer application improves balance and activity of daily living in individuals with stroke: a randomized controlled trial. PLoS One. **17**(11), e0277870 (2022)
22. Moreno-Ligero, M., et al.: mHealth impact on gait and dynamic balance outcomes in neurorehabilitation: systematic review and meta-analysis. J. Med. Syst. **47**(1), 75 (2023)
23. Grau-Pellicer, M., et al.: Impact of mHealth technology on adherence to healthy PA after stroke: a randomized study. Top. Stroke Rehabil. **27**(5), 354–368 (2020)
24. McGarrigle, L., Boulton, E., Todd, C.: Map the apps: a rapid review of digital approaches to support the engagement of older adults in strength and balance exercises. BMC Geriatr. **20**(1), 483 (2020)
25. Skelton, D.A., et al.: Prevention of Falls Network Europe: a thematic network aimed at introducing good practice in effective falls prevention across Europe. Eur. J. Ageing. **1**(1), 89–94 (2004)
26. Sousa, C.V., et al.: A systematic review and meta-analysis of the effect of active video games on postural balance. Arch. Phys. Med. Rehabil. **104**(4), 631–644 (2023)
27. Primack, B.A., et al.: Role of video games in improving health-related outcomes: a systematic review. Am. J. Prev. Med. **42**(6), 630–638 (2012)
28. Ma, W., et al.: Physical activity, sedentary behavior, and risk of coronavirus disease 2019. Am. J. Med. **136**(6), 568–576.e3 (2023)
29. Wu, J., Loprinzi, P.D., Ren, Z.: The rehabilitative effects of virtual reality games on balance performance among children with cerebral palsy: a meta-analysis of randomized controlled trials. Int. J. Environ. Res. Public Health. **16**(21) (2019)
30. Taylor, L.M., et al.: Active video games for improving physical performance measures in older people: a meta-analysis. J. Geriatr. Phys. Ther. **41**(2), 108–123 (2018)
31. Hocking, D.R., et al.: Do active video games improve motor function in people with developmental disabilities? A meta-analysis of randomized controlled trials. Arch. Phys. Med. Rehabil. **100**(4), 769–781 (2019)
32. Chen, Y., et al.: Comparison between the effects of exergame intervention and traditional physical training on improving balance and fall prevention in healthy older adults: a systematic review and meta-analysis. J. Neuroeng. Rehabil. **18**(1), 164 (2021)
33. Wang, S., et al.: Can recovery foot placement affect older adults' slip-fall severity? Ann. Biomed. Eng. **45**(8), 1941–1948 (2017)

34. Pijnappels, M., Bobbert, M.F., van Dieën, J.H.: Push-off reactions in recovery after tripping discriminate young subjects, older non-fallers and older fallers. Gait Posture. **21**(4), 388–394 (2005)
35. Okubo, Y., et al.: Effect of reactive balance training involving repeated slips and trips on balance recovery among older adults: a blinded randomized controlled trial. J. Gerontol. A. **74**(9), 1489–1496 (2019)
36. Batcir, S., et al.: Characteristics of step responses following varying magnitudes of unexpected lateral perturbations during standing among older people - a cross-sectional laboratory-based study. BMC Geriatr. **22**(1), 400 (2022)
37. Mille, M.L., et al.: Age-dependent differences in lateral balance recovery through protective stepping. Clin. Biomech. (Bristol). **20**(6), 607–616 (2005)
38. Maeda, Y., et al.: A preliminary study of static and dynamic standing balance and risk of falling in an independent elderly population with a particular focus on the limit of stability test. J. Phys. Ther. Sci. **23**(5), 803–806 (2011)
39. Maeda, Y., et al.: Effect of load change on foot arch in different positions—assessment of foot arch using a motion analysis system and a Caliper—goniometer system—. J. Phys. Ther. Sci. **24**(5), 435–441 (2012)
40. Maeda, Y., et al.: Dynamic postural adjustments in stance in response to translational perturbation in presence of visual and somatosensory disturbance. J. Med. Biol. Eng. **34**, 333–340 (2014)
41. Maeda, Y., et al.: Age-related changes in dynamic postural control ability in the presence of sensory perturbation. J. Med. Biol. Eng. **35**(1), 86–93 (2015)
42. Maeda, Y., Sudo, D., Shimotori, D.: Different effects of 12-week speed or accuracy training on obstacle-crossing foot motion in healthy elderly. Int. J. Environ. Res. Public Health. **19**(8), 4596 (2022)
43. Maeda, Y., Sudo, D., Shimotori, D.: Age-related changes in accuracy and speed of lateral crossing motion: focus on stepping from leaning position. Int. J. Environ. Res. Public Health. **19**(15), 9056 (2022)
44. Tanaka, T., Noriyasu, S., Ino, S., Ifukube, T., Nakata, M.: Objective method to determine the contribution of the great toe to standing balance and preliminary observations of age-related effects. IEEE Trans. Rehabil. Eng. **4**(2), 84–90 (1996)
45. Lord, S.R., Clark, R.D., Webster, I.W.: Physiological factors associated with falls in an elderly population. J. Am. Geriatr. Soc. **39**(12), 1194–1200 (1991). https://doi.org/10.1111/j.1532-5415.1991.tb03574.x
46. Maki, B.E., Holliday, P.J., Topper, A.K.: Fear of falling and postural performance in the elderly. J. Gerontol. **46**(4), M123–M131 (1991). https://doi.org/10.1093/geronj/46.4.m123
47. Priplata, A.A., Niemi, J.B., Harry, J.D., Lipsitz, L.A., Collins, J.J.: Vibrating insoles and balance control in elderly people. Lancet. **362**(9390), 1123–1124 (2003). https://doi.org/10.1016/S0140-6736(03)14470-4
48. Peterka, R.J.: Sensorimotor integration in human postural control. J. Neurophysiol. **88**(3), 1097–1118 (2002). https://doi.org/10.1152/jn.2002.88.3.1097
49. Tanaka, T., Shirogane, S., Izumi, T., Ino, S., Ifukube, T.: The effect of brief moving vibratory stimulation on the feet for postural control in a comparison study. Phys. Occup. Ther. Geriatr. **24**(1):1–23 (2005)
50. Tanaka, T., Shirogane, S., Maeda, Y., Sugihara, S., Miyasaka, T., Kido, S., Izumi, T.: Effectiveness of a new combined system, using a force plate and vibratory stimulation device for balance training in patients with stroke. In: Proceedings of 1st International Conference on Applied Bionics and Biomechanics ICABB-2010, Venezia, Italy (2010)

51. Tanaka, T., Maeda, Y., Miura, T.: Effects of tactile sensory stimulation training of the trunk and sole on standing balance ability in older adults: a randomized controlled trial. J. Funct. Morphol. Kinesiol. **10**(1), 96 (2025). https://doi.org/10.3390/jfmk10010096
52. Tanaka, T., Kojima, S., Takeda, H., Ino, S., Ifukube, T.: The influence of moving auditory stimuli on standing balance in healthy adults with aging. Ergonomics. **44**(15), 1403–1412 (2001)

Chapter 6
Supporting Mobility for the Elderly and Persons with Disabilities 1

Satoshi Shirogane and Toshiaki Tanaka

Abstract Wheelchairs are essential assistive devices that support mobility and independence in both older adults and individuals with disabilities. Although their history dates back to ancient times, modern designs incorporating lightweight materials and foldable structures emerged in the early twentieth century. Today, wheelchairs have diversified into specialized models for sports and caregiving, with electric wheelchairs significantly reducing physical strain and enabling greater social participation.

In Japan, public funding and policy initiatives have played a crucial role in wheelchair provision. Since the enactment of the Act on Welfare of Physically Disabled Persons in 1949, various assistive devices have been subsidized to enhance the independence and quality of daily life. The scope of financial support has expanded over time, including the introduction of electric wheelchairs in 1989 and advanced postural support systems in 1990.

Despite long-standing public support, the effectiveness of assistive device provisions remains insufficiently analyzed. The research report tracking 1997–2023 trends revealed a decline in manual wheelchair subsidies, largely due to the Long-Term Care Insurance Act promoting rental-based distribution. Electric wheelchair provisions remain relatively stable but show a gradual decline. Understanding these policy trends is key to optimizing future welfare programs.

Ensuring the mechanical safety and effectiveness of wheelchairs is crucial for user confidence, injury prevention, and functional optimization. Given that a wheelchair is essentially an extension of the user's body, mechanical failures can lead to serious injuries, necessitating continuous assessment and improvements in design and materials.

S. Shirogane
Clinical Evaluation Section, Department of Assistive Technology, Research Institute, National Rehabilitation Center for Persons with Disabilities, Tokorozawa, Japan
e-mail: shirogane-satoshi@rehab.go.jp

T. Tanaka (✉)
Research Center for Advanced Science and Technology/Institute of Gerontology, The University of Tokyo, Tokyo, Japan
e-mail: t.tanaka@iog.u-tokyo.ac.jp; tanaka@bfp.rcast.u-tokyo.ac.jp

T. Tanaka (ed.), *Inclusive and Barrier-Free Designs for Rehabilitation Engineering*,
https://doi.org/10.1007/978-981-95-5783-7_6

Industry standards such as the ISO and JIS help regulate wheelchair durability, but evolving user needs demand ongoing evaluations. For example, excessive force exerted by users with cerebral palsy or stroke-related hemiplegia can lead to wheelchair structural failure, thereby posing risks. Studies on foot and head support have quantified mechanical loads, revealing that foot support forces can reach 134% of body weight, while head support loads during spastic episodes can reach 88.3% of body weight.

Beyond safety, the compatibility between wheelchairs and users affects comfort and pressure ulcer risk. While the pressure distribution is widely measured, shear force remains difficult to assess owing to sensor limitations. To address this, researchers have developed thin, flexible shear force sensors that can successfully visualize force variations during posture shifts. Future research should refine measurement techniques to enhance scientific wheelchair-user assessments and ensure optimal adaptation for assistive mobility devices.

With the progression of population aging, accidents involving wheelchair use by elderly individuals with cognitive impairments are increasing. In this study, we developed a multisensory alert system to support safe wheelchair operation and training. The system was gradually improved by incorporating sensors on the brakes and foot supports, as well as combining visual, auditory, and vibratory feedback. In the final stage, visual guidance through visual stimuli was also introduced. The system was evaluated with elderly individuals who had cerebrovascular disorders and moderate cognitive impairment, and the results showed a reduction in operational errors and task completion time under the condition combining visual, auditory, and vibratory stimuli. This system is expected to be useful for future clinical applications and for use in home and institutional settings, serving as an effective aid for learning safe wheelchair operation.

6.1 Wheelchairs Supporting the Mobility of Individuals with Disabilities and Older Adults

6.1.1 Wheelchairs: Their Importance and Technological Advancements

A wheelchair is one of the most essential assistive devices that supports the mobility and daily lives of older adults and individuals with disabilities. Their effective utilization enables them to engage in activities that were previously challenging or inaccessible.

The history of wheelchairs dates back to ancient times. However, the introduction of lightweight materials and foldable designs began in the early twentieth century, when the foundation of modern wheelchair technology was established relatively recently.

Wheelchair designs have expanded beyond traditional manual models to include specialized variants tailored for sports, caregiving, and other specific applications.

Furthermore, the development and widespread adoption of electric wheelchairs have significantly reduced the physical strain associated with mobility, thereby enhancing opportunities for social participation among individuals who depend on such devices.

In recent years, electric wheelchairs have undergone substantial technological advancements, with efforts to integrate features such as obstacle detection for collision avoidance, autonomous driving capabilities, and real-time usage-monitoring systems. Such innovations have evolved at an accelerated pace. To enhance the practical utility of these wheelchairs for individuals with disabilities and older adults and to facilitate their seamless and proactive integration into daily life, it is imperative to sustain and further advance research in welfare engineering and rehabilitation engineering.

6.1.2 Public Funding and Policy Support for Wheelchairs in Japan

The provision and support for mobility-assistive devices, such as wheelchairs, for individuals with disabilities have advanced through various national support policies and initiatives led by the World Health Organization (WHO).

Japan is an economically developed country that has long provided publicly funded wheelchairs to individuals whose need for mobility assistance is recognized as essential for employment and improvement of daily life. In 1949, the Act on the Welfare of Physically Disabled Persons was enacted to promote independence and socioeconomic participation among individuals with physical disabilities. As part of the country's welfare services, assistive devices such as wheelchairs and seating support chairs have become available.

Subsequent amendments to the legislation expanded the scope of support. In 1989, electric wheelchairs were added to a list of publicly funded assistive devices. In 1990, higher-functionality postural support devices were introduced to accommodate cases in which basic low-cost seating support chairs were insufficient.

The number of individuals in Japan with some form of disability is estimated to be approximately 11.6 million, accounting for approximately 9.2% of the total population [1]. This includes 4.36 million individuals with physical disabilities, 1.094 million with intellectual disabilities, and 6.148 million with mental disabilities, with the overall number of people with disabilities reportedly increasing. Although mobility-assistive devices such as wheelchairs are primarily required by individuals with physical disabilities, Japan's aging population has further heightened the importance of these assistive technologies.

6.1.3 Public Support for Wheelchairs and Mobility-Assistance Devices in Japan

However, the actual status of publicly funded assistive device provisions for individuals with disabilities has not been thoroughly examined, and the effectiveness of public funding remains unclear. Therefore, we analyzed the trends in government-funded wheelchair distribution from 1997 to 2016 based on the Report on Social Welfare Administration and Services [2], a statistical resource published annually by the Ministry of Health, Labour and Welfare of Japan [3]. This report quantitatively captures administrative practices across prefectures, designated cities, and core cities following the implementation of various social welfare laws, including the Act on Welfare of Physically Disabled Persons and the Child Welfare Act. Figures 6.1 and 6.2 illustrate the yearly number of newly approved wheelchairs and electric wheelchair provisions, incorporating the latest data from 2023 into the previously visualized dataset.

In 1999, publicly funded manual wheelchair provisions exceeded 80,000 units; however, the number declined sharply, following a continuous downward trend until 2023 (Fig. 6.1). This reduction is largely attributed to the implementation of Japan's Long-Term Care Insurance Act, which expanded rental-based wheelchair distribution for elderly individuals. In Japan's assistive device subsidy system, publicly funded provisions are subordinate to other available programs, implying that alternative support mechanisms take precedence. Additionally, the sharp decline in provisions in 2006 was largely attributable to the revision of the Act on Support

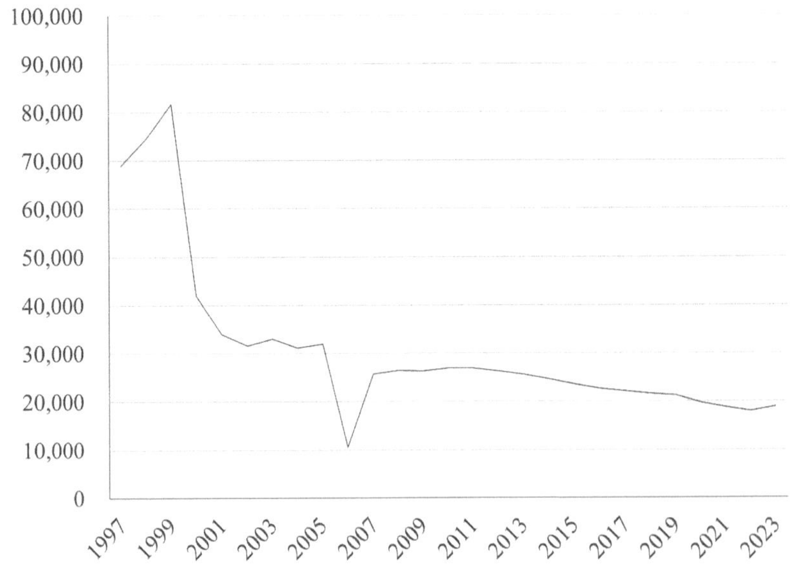

Fig. 6.1 The trend in the number of wheelchair purchase subsidies provided under Japan's public system

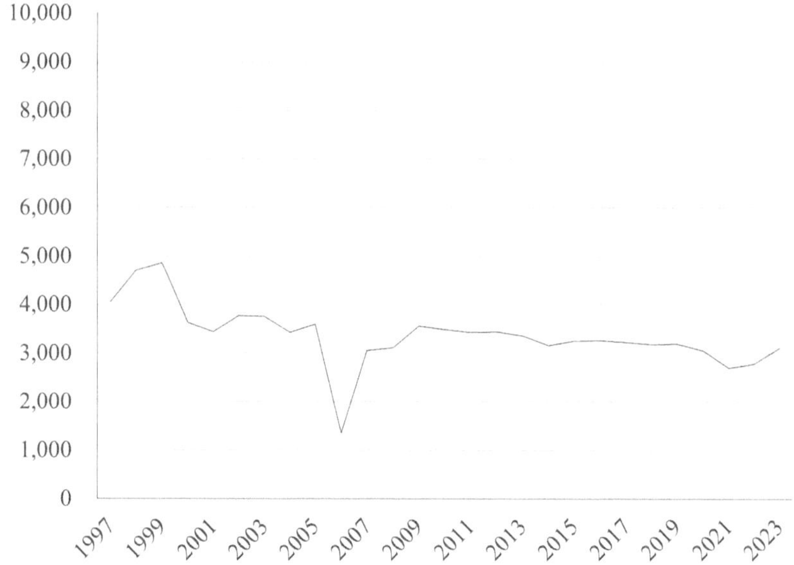

Fig. 6.2 The trend in the number of powered wheelchair purchase subsidies provided under Japan's public system

for Persons with Disabilities. Because of this legislative change, the collection of statistical data was restricted to the period from October to March, leading to an apparent decrease in the total number of provisions.

The annual number of publicly funded electric wheelchairs has remained relatively stable at 3000–5000 units, although a gradual decline has been observed (Fig. 6.2). The proportion of electric wheelchair provisions relative to manual wheelchairs is approximately 1:10. The impact of long-term care insurance policies appears minimal for electric wheelchairs, possibly because of their limited use among elderly individuals. Regarding the sharp decline in 2006, the underlying cause was similar to that of manual wheelchair use.

It should be noted that these figures represent the number of newly approved subsidy cases each year rather than the total number of users. Wheelchairs and other assistive devices are assigned a standard durability period during which continued use is generally expected. However, if an individual's physical condition or living environment changes, the required type or specifications of wheelchair may also change, necessitating modifications or replacements before the standard period expires.

In addition, Japan has a public long-term care insurance program that targets elderly individuals (65 years or older) and those aged 40–65 years with designated medical conditions. This system provides rental-based wheelchair provisions, with approximately 800,000 units lost by 2023 [4]. Figure 6.3 illustrates the historical trends in wheelchair rentals, showing a consistent upward trajectory that likely contributed to the decline in direct government-funded provisions. While

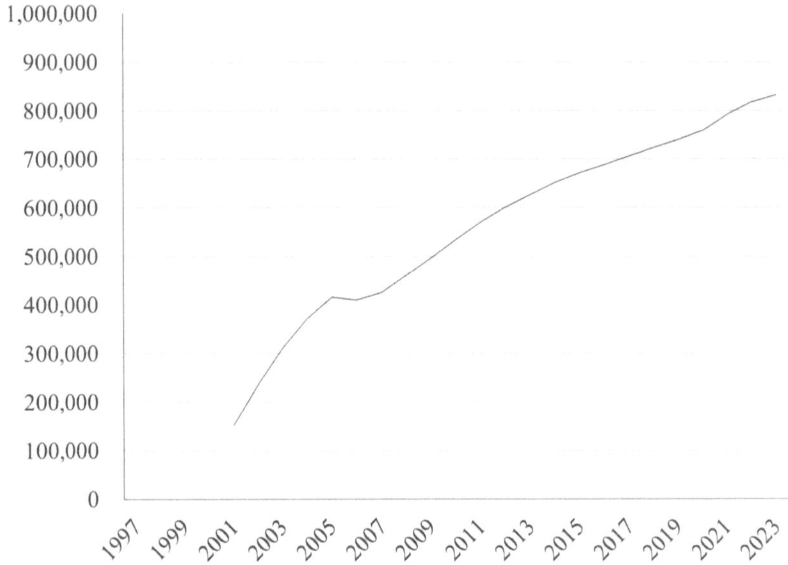

Fig. 6.3 The trend in the number of wheelchair rentals under Japan's long-term care insurance system

rental-based wheelchairs lack the customization potential of individually manufactured units, model adjustments and component modifications allow adaptability to various user needs. If the standard rental models prove insufficient, custom production through assistive device subsidies remains an option.

Understanding public provision trends for wheelchairs and mobility assistance devices is crucial for evaluating policy effectiveness and guiding future system improvements. By analyzing usage patterns and statistical trends, policymakers can enhance accessibility and user-friendliness more effectively. Furthermore, insights into Japan's welfare model may serve as a valuable reference for international public support systems aimed at optimizing wheelchair distribution.

6.2 Mechanical Safety and Effectiveness Evaluation of Wheelchairs

6.2.1 Ensuring the Safety and Utility of Wheelchairs

To ensure that wheelchairs serve as practical and reliable tools in society, safety must be guaranteed. For users, a wheelchair effectively becomes an extension of their body, meaning that any failure or malfunction can lead to severe injury. The structural components of a wheelchair must possess sufficient mechanical strength, and considerable effort has been devoted to optimizing materials, design, and manufacturing techniques. However, with gradual changes in social environments and usage conditions, continuous assessments and improvements are necessary.

As wheelchair designs have evolved to include a wider range of structures and functionalities, the need for effectiveness evaluation has also increased. Ultimately, the effectiveness of a wheelchair is closely linked to its users' quality of life (QOL), necessitating assessments tailored to individual characteristics and intended purposes. For instance, when a user selects a wheelchair or when a model is designated for public support programs, scientific data on effectiveness are essential to inform decision-making.

Thus, ensuring the safety and effectiveness of wheelchairs and related assistive devices, such as posture support systems, is vital in building a society in which individuals with disabilities can use these technologies with confidence. Ongoing research in these areas is crucial to foster a supportive and functional environment.

6.2.2 Research on the Mechanical Strength Required for Wheelchairs

Industry standards, such as those set by the International Organization for Standardization, are essential for ensuring product safety and are regularly updated to reflect advancements in disability analysis, societal shifts, and technological progress. The ISO has issued multiple wheelchair-related standards, many of which have been adopted by the Japanese Industrial Standards (JIS). With the continuous introduction of new features and devices in wheelchair technology and evolving user environments, ongoing evaluations are crucial.

For example, individuals with cerebral palsy or stroke-induced hemiplegia may experience involuntary intense muscle contractions, exerting excessive force on wheelchair structures. Several cases of wheelchair failure owing to extreme loads have been reported in Japan. Because such damage poses a serious injury risk to users, minimizing its occurrence is crucial. To improve safety, existing testing methods and guidelines for components subjected to high mechanical stress must be reviewed. However, few studies have quantitatively measured these forces, and data on specific load values remain limited.

To bridge these gaps, we conducted quantitative load measurements to assess testing methods and reference thresholds for mitigating user risk. Our study specifically examined foot and head support.

Foot Support Load Measurements

Foot supports were tested according to ISO standards [5], which specify the application of a vertical load to assess the mechanical resistance (Fig. 6.4). The Ministry of Health, Labour and Welfare of Japan guidelines [6] set testing thresholds based on user weight: $\leq$25 kg: 250 N, $\leq$50 kg: 500 N, $\leq$75 kg: 750 N, $\leq$100 kg: 1000 N.

Measurements were conducted on three individuals with severe spastic cerebral palsy (male, 10 s; male, 30 s; female, 40 s) [7]. The load assessment was performed

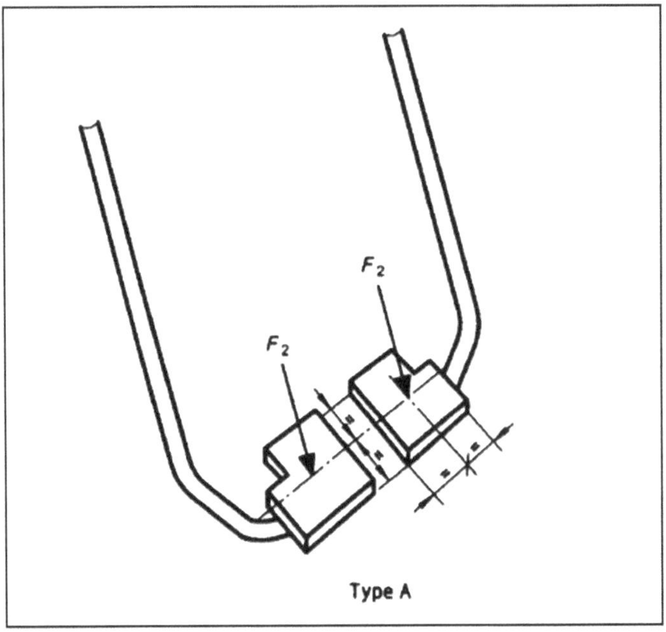

Fig. 6.4 Foot support test method of the International Organization for Standardization [5]

Fig. 6.5 Experimental setting; PC, personal computer; Fz, vertical force on the foot support; Fx and Fy, horizontal forces on the foot support. Reproduced with permission of the Society of Physical Therapy Science. [7]

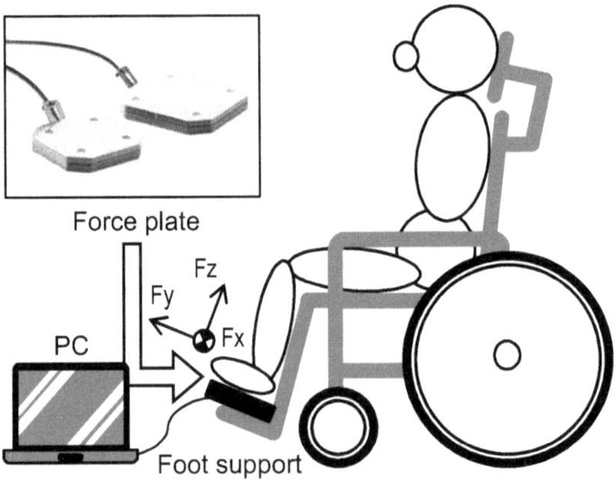

using two portable force plates placed between the users' feet and the foot support structures (Fig. 6.5). The variations in the vertical and horizontal forces over time are shown in Fig. 6.6. Subjects 1 and 3 showed increases in both vertical and horizontal forces as the load intensified, whereas subject 2 exhibited no horizontal force increase, displaying a distinct pattern. The maximum recorded load was 525 N (instantaneous), reaching 134% of body weight [7].

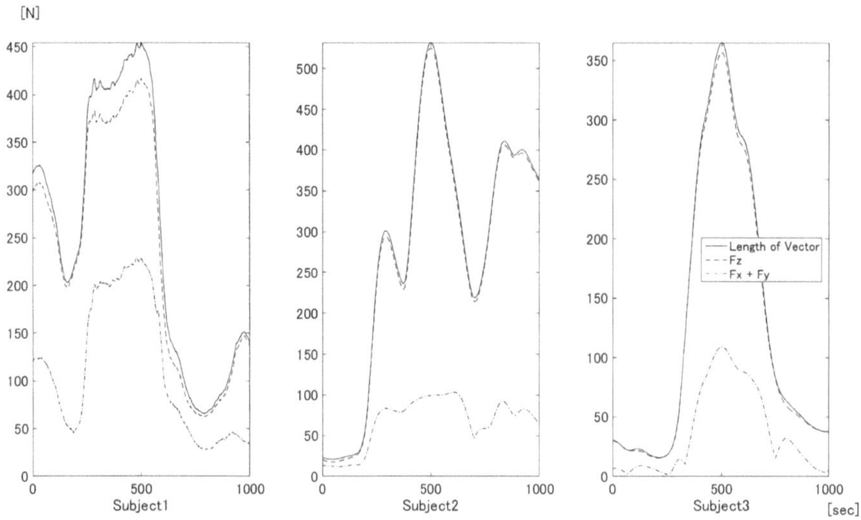

Fig. 6.6 Temporal changes in the load vector and vertical and horizontal components. Reproduced with permission of the Society of Physical Therapy Science. [7]

Head Support Load Measurements
A 30-year-old male with severe spastic cerebral palsy [8], presenting tetraplegia and using a Panda Seating System equipped with head support (R82-81483, R82). The subject required near-total assistance for daily activities, and his physical therapist reported frequent, intense spastic episodes that exerted excessive force on head support.

To quantify mechanical stress, a strain gauge (KFG-5-120-C1-11L1M2R, Kyowa Electronic Instruments) was affixed to the head support column using a specialized adhesive (CC33A, Kyowa Electronic Instruments, Japan).

The results indicated that forces applied during spastic episodes reached up to 88.3% of the body weight (Fig. 6.7), highlighting the need for further evaluation and structural reinforcement of head support components in wheelchairs designed for individuals with severe motor impairments.

6.2.3 *Research on Wheelchair Compatibility with the Human Body*

Effective and safe wheelchair use depends on the optimal compatibility between the user's body and assistive device. Insufficient compatibility not only diminishes the wheelchair's functional benefits but also increases the risk of secondary injuries, such as pressure ulcers. In clinical practice, specialists carefully select and adjust wheelchairs and cushions based on the user's physical condition and the daily living

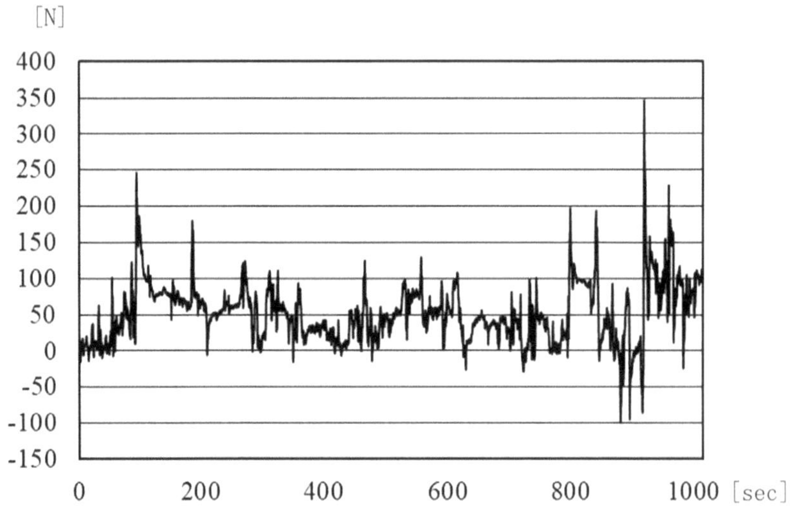

Fig. 6.7 Partial measurement data from strain gauge. Reproduced with permission of the Rigakuryoho Kagaku. [8]

environment. However, the current assessment methods rely heavily on expert judgment, professional intuition, and user feedback, underscoring the need for objective measurement tools to evaluate compatibility more scientifically.

Development of a Thin and Flexible Sensor

The two primary objective indicators of wheelchair-user compatibility are pressure distribution and shear force. However, measuring the shear force remains challenging owing to sensor design limitations and scarcity of available data. Conventional shear force sensors tend to be bulky or excessively thick, which hinders their practical applications. Thus, the development of thin flexible sensors that can be seamlessly integrated between the user and wheelchair is essential.

To address this challenge, we developed a shear force sensor composed entirely of soft materials, including flexible film electrodes (bendable but nonstretchable), elastic rubber, and liquid electrolytes (Fig. 6.8) [9]. After stabilization, the sensor exhibited resistance to temperature and pressure while supporting extended film-based wiring, making it well suited for real-world applications. Subsequently, this shear force sensor was integrated with a pressure sensor, enabling three-axis force measurements at contact points [10]. Using this combined sensor system, we conducted continuous quantitative shear force measurements on the wheelchair seat surfaces.

Preliminary Evaluation of Postural History Effects on Shear Force

The shear force acting on the buttocks may not be solely determined by the posture at the time of measurement but could also be influenced by prior postural transitions, a phenomenon referred to as the postural history effect. This suggests that even if a

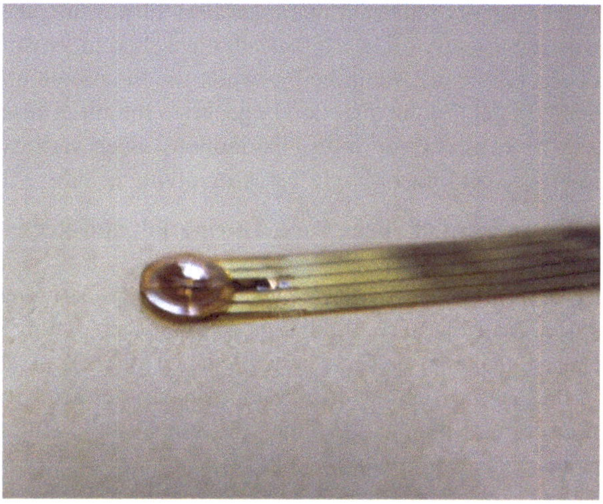

Fig. 6.8 A thin and flexible shear force sensor developed by our research group

subject assumes the same posture at the measurement point, the sequence of preceding postures may affect the distribution and magnitude of the shear force.

For example, when transitioning from a laterally tilted posture to a neutral seated position, residual forces from the previous lateral tilt may influence the shear force distribution at the buttocks. Similarly, differences in shear stress accumulation can arise depending on whether a neutral posture follows a forward-leaning or backward-leaning posture. If these variations are consistently observed, they highlight the potential importance of incorporating postural history into shear force evaluations, rather than assessing each posture in isolation.

To explore these effects, a sensor was embedded into a cushion at the ischial tuberosity of one side to measure shear force under different postural conditions [11]. The measurements were conducted on a subject seated in a wheelchair who actively tilted their own torso forward, backward, right, and left before returning to a neutral posture. The results showed no significant differences in shear force along the anteroposterior axis (sagittal plane) based on the prior postures. However, the shear force along the mediolateral axis (frontal plane) exhibited notable variations. Specifically, when transitioning through a laterally tilted posture, there was a tendency for shear force directed inward to increase more than when transitioning through an anterior-posterior tilted posture.

While this study was conducted on a single subject, the findings suggest the possible effects of postural history on shear force distribution under specific conditions. This phenomenon could have important implications for wheelchair seating ergonomics and pressure ulcer prevention.

Shear Force Variations in Different Seated Postures

To investigate the general characteristics of the shear force acting on the buttocks, shear force measurements were conducted on nine healthy subjects in different seated postures [12]. A shear force sensor embedded in a cushion was installed in a wheelchair, and the subjects actively tilted their torso forward, backward, left, and right, maintaining each posture for several seconds.

The results indicated that regardless of posture, shear force directed posteriorly was consistently observed beneath the ischial tuberosities in healthy subjects seated in a wheelchair. Additionally, when the torso was tilted laterally, the shear force tended to act in the direction opposite to the tilt. These findings suggest a potential pattern in the shear force distribution under various seated postures, providing reference data for future research involving healthy subjects.

Measurement of Shear Force During Tilt and Recline Using a Multipoint Shear Force Measurement System
To achieve enhanced three-axis shear force measurements, we developed a sensor system capable of multipoint detection by integrating pressure measurements with shear force analysis. This system enables the visualization of continuous variations in pressure and shear force at the contact interface between the wheelchair and the user during tilting and reclining movements, allowing for a quantifiable assessment of wheelchair-user compatibility [13].

For practical validation, sensors were installed on the seat and back support of a powered wheelchair to measure the shear force during the tilt and recline operations. As a preliminary step before human testing, we conducted experiments using a humanoid dummy covered with a soft urethane sponge, allowing the tactile confirmation of landmark points. The dummy was positioned in an electric wheelchair with sensors attached, as shown in Fig. 6.9, to record shear force variations during tilt and recline.

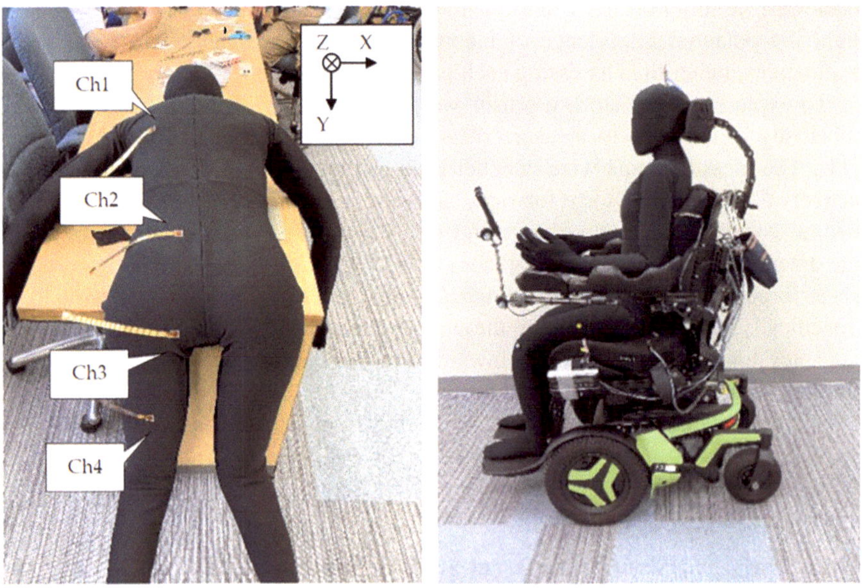

Fig. 6.9 Experimental setup. On the left, the dummy is shown with the sensor attached. To facilitate understanding of the sensor's placement, the image depicts the state before fabric attachment. On the right, the dummy is seated in an electric wheelchair, with multiple markers affixed to both the dummy and the wheelchair to monitor posture

Time-dependent variations in shear force along different axes are illustrated in Fig. 6.10 for reclining and Fig. 6.11 for tilting; the force direction is defined as positive toward the feet and negative toward the head along the vertical axis and positive inward and negative outward along the lateral axis. Across repeated trials, the observed force trajectories remained highly consistent, confirming the stability and repeatability of shear force measurements. This system is expected to provide valuable insights into the dynamics of the contact interface between the wheelchair and the user's body during posture adjustments such as tilting and reclining.

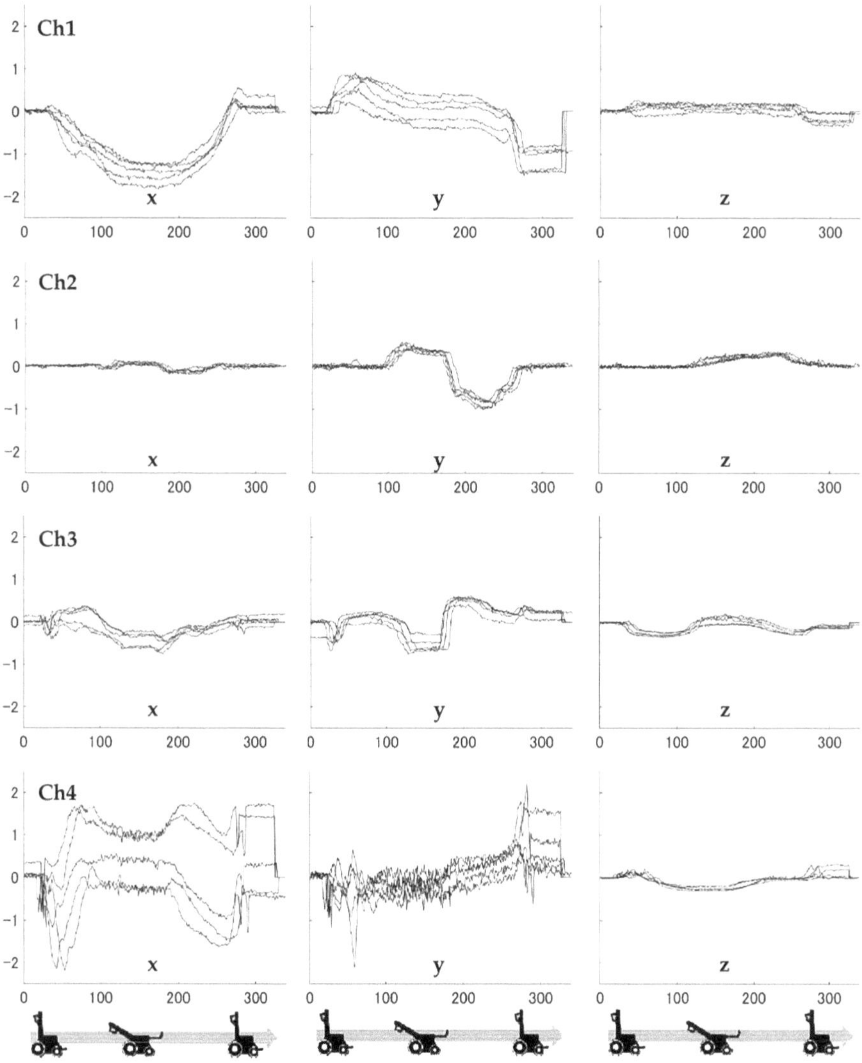

Fig. 6.10 Load values for the three axes at each sensor (recline pattern)

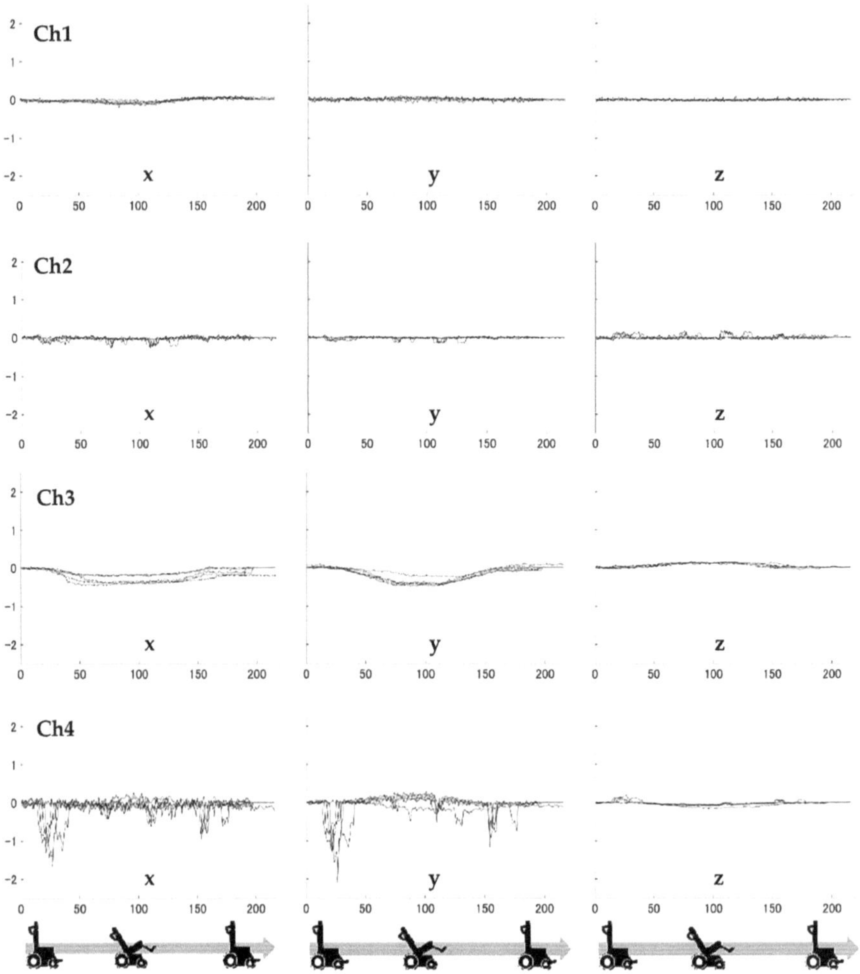

Fig. 6.11 Load values for the three axes at each sensor (tilting pattern)

Future Perspectives on Shear Force Quantification in Wheelchair Users
Quantifying the shear force in wheelchair users remains a challenge, and comprehensive implementation is still limited. However, the ability to conduct such assessments plays a crucial role in the scientific evaluation of wheelchair-user compatibility, highlighting the need for continued research and technological advancements in this field.

6.3 Alert System for Wheelchair Operation: Training, Support, and Assistive Devices

6.3.1 Background

As the Japanese population ages, the proportion of elderly people with dementia and other forms of higher brain dysfunction is increasing rapidly. Consequently, incidents related to mobility and transfers, especially falls and mishandling during wheelchair use, have become serious issues. According to a 2010 report by the Ministry of Health, Labour and Welfare, approximately 2.8 million people aged 65 and over had dementia, and this number is expected to exceed 4.8 million by 2025 [14]. Against this backdrop, developing equipment that supports the safe and independent mobility of the elderly has become a pressing social issue. Although traditional wheelchairs are easy to operate, users with cognitive impairments often make operating errors, which can lead to serious accidents. Pellichero et al. (2021) reported that cognitive function influences the ability to operate personal mobility devices (PMDs) and emphasized the importance of evaluating spatial cognition and attention functions [15]. Furthermore, Hou et al. (2024) highlighted the future potential of technological support, noting that Internet of Things (IoT)-enabled autonomous wheelchairs allow for vital sign monitoring and remote assistance [16].

6.3.2 Development Process and Purpose

The development of the wheelchair alert system (Figs. 6.12, 6.13, 6.14, and 6.15) was conducted in multiple stages [17]. In the first stage, a prototype was designed that used sensors to detect brake operation and foot support position. This prototype provided alerts via light and voice. This prototype employed wired connections and emphasized immediate feedback to user actions. In the second stage, circuit adjustments were made to reduce misdetection rates of the sensors, and vibrotactile feedback via vibration motors was introduced. Clinical observations during this phase revealed misuse patterns among users with cognitive impairments and led to design improvements. The third stage involved miniaturizing and making the system wireless and adding a visual guidance function using a head-mounted display (HMD) to support users with visual perceptual impairments. Based on these development phases, the aim of this study was to support learning to operate a wheelchair and prevent operational errors through a system that integrates multiple sensory stimuli.

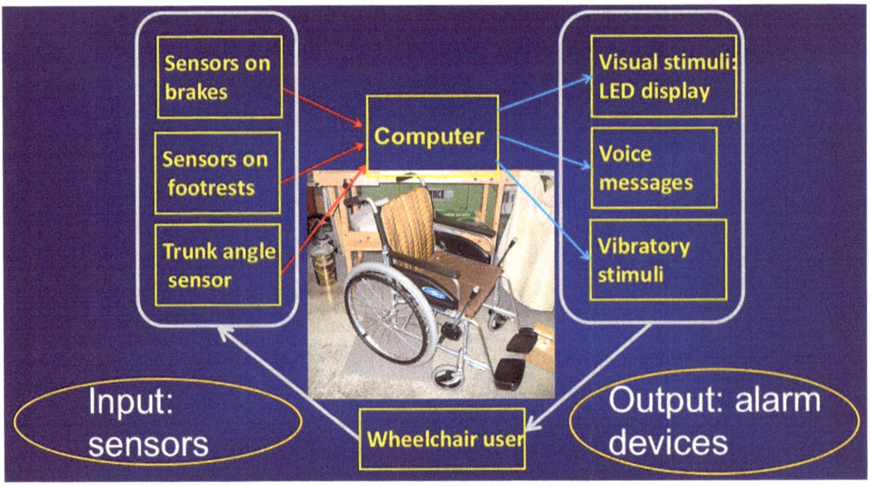

Fig. 6.12 Information flow in the new alert wheelchair system. (© Springer Nature. Reproduced under the publisher's author reuse policy [17])

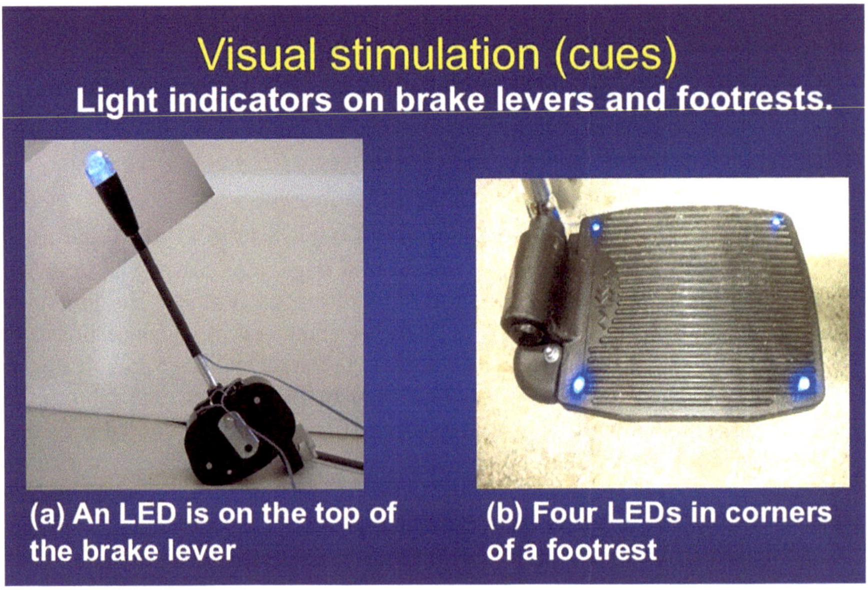

Fig. 6.13 LEDs indicate the place of next action by light stimulation. (© Springer Nature. Reproduced under the publisher's author reuse policy [17])

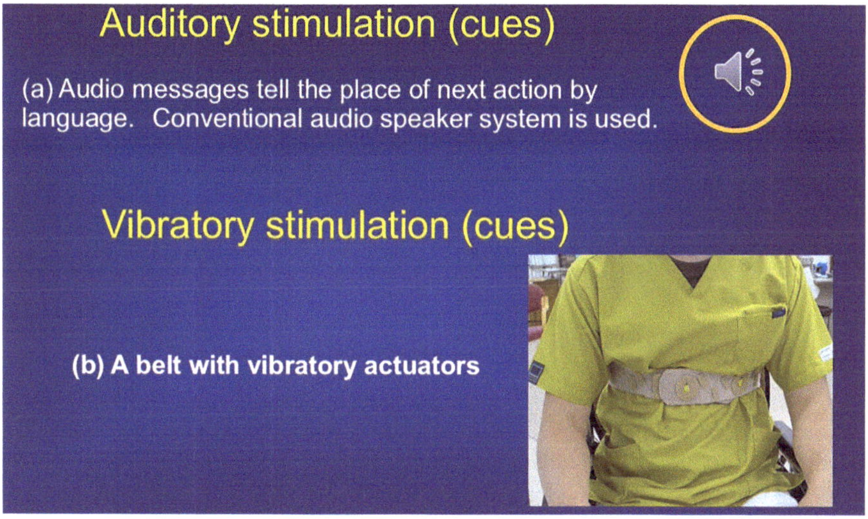

Fig. 6.14 Auditory and vibratory stimili devices for alarm system. (© Springer Nature. Reproduced under the publisher's author reuse policy [17])

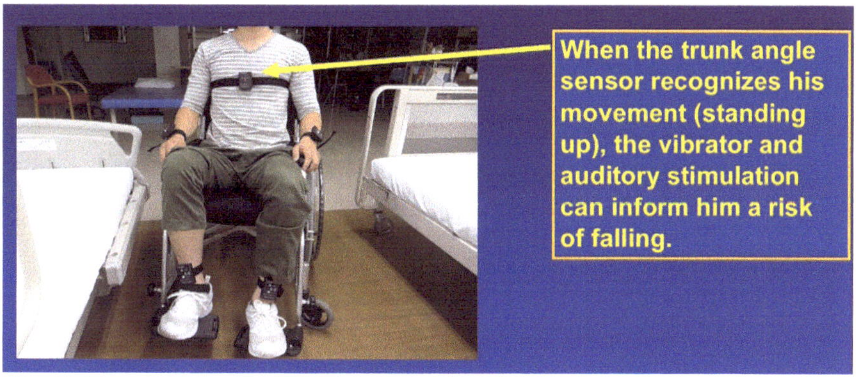

Fig. 6.15 Wireless trunk angle sensors for detecting trunk movements in relation to falling. (© Springer Nature. Reproduced under the publisher's author reuse policy [17])

6.3.3 Methods

Based on the study design described in ref. [17], eight patients with cerebrovascular disorders and moderate to severe cognitive impairment (mean age: 73 years) were selected as subjects. Their Mini-Mental State Examination (MMSE) scores ranged from 20 to 24, indicating mild to moderate cognitive impairment. The system used a PIC microcontroller as the control board and combined the following sensors and output devices (Figs. 6.12, 6.13, 6.14, and 6.15): (1) a contact sensor on the brake lever, (2) an open/close sensor on the foot support, (3) a seating sensor under the seat, (4) a tilt sensor on the backrest, (5) an LED for visual stimuli, (6) a speaker for voice prompts, and (7) a vibration motor for tactile feedback. Experiments were conducted under four conditions: normal, visual + vibration, auditory and+ vibration, and visual + auditory + vibration. Evaluation metrics included operation time, number of operational errors, number of stops, and task completion rate before standing. Actions were recorded via video motion analysis and evaluated by multiple physical therapists. Additional experiments were conducted using an HMD-based visual guidance condition for subjects with visual perceptual impairment.

6.3.4 Results

The most notable improvement in wheelchair operation was observed under the visual, auditory, and vibration stimulation condition (Fig. 6.16), with a reduction in operational errors across all participants. Operation time was also reduced, and motion analysis showed improved compliance with preparatory procedures for standing actions. Figure 6.16 shows that the average number of operational errors under the normal (no stimulus) condition was 12 and was reduced to 2 under the visual, auditory, and vibration stimulation condition. Using the HMD to provide visual information to users with visual perceptual impairments tended to be effective for subjects exhibiting spatial neglect. However, some participants experienced delays due to a limited visual field or unfamiliarity with the device. Signal

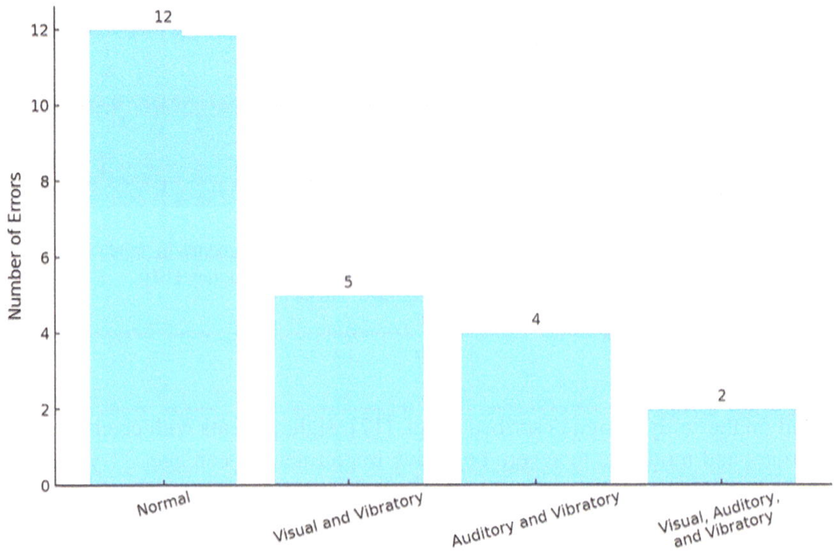

Fig. 6.16 Comparison of error frequency by stimulation condition. (© Springer Nature. Reproduced under the publisher's author reuse policy [17])

processing delays from the sensors and differences in recognizing voice guidance were also observed and identified as areas for improvement in the future.

6.3.5 Discussion

Using multisensory integration involving visual, auditory, and tactile stimuli was highly effective in supporting wheelchair operation for individuals with cognitive impairments. Subjects who did not adequately respond to visual information alone were able to better understand the correct procedures when audio and vibration cues were combined. These results align with those of Pellichero et al. (2021), who emphasized the relationship between operational behavior and attention function [15]. Furthermore, integrating this system with the autonomous technology proposed by Hou et al. (2024) could enable more advanced accident prevention and health monitoring in the future [16]. However, significant individual differences in HMD usability were observed, and visual guidance was burdensome in some cases. Therefore, prior assessment and training are essential.

6.3.6 Conclusion

This study confirmed the effectiveness of the wheelchair alert system for elderly individuals with cognitive impairments. It is expected to be clinically applicable for operation training and ensuring safety. Moving forward, efforts will focus on improving adaptability to diverse usage environments, enhancing sensor performance, and refining the user interface to promote broader adoption in home and institutional settings.

In the context of inclusive design studies concerning this issue, this alert system, designed for repeated wheelchair operation training for elderly individuals and persons with cognitive impairments, enables users to engage in training independently, potentially leading to improved operational skills. However, conducting an adequate assessment of the user's level of disability and ensuring that elderly and disabled users are not confused or overwhelmed by the alert system constitute an essential aspect of inclusive design research. Evaluating and analyzing the environmental conditions that the user will face after discharge, and incorporating these factors into the design of this system through discussions involving the user and their family, are also of great importance.

References

1. Cabinet Office Japan: FY2024 annual report on government measures for persons with disabilities. https://www8.cao.go.jp/shougai/whitepaper/index-w.html (in Japanese)
2. Shirogane, S.: Provision of public funding for wheelchairs and postural support devices in Japan. J. Phys. Ther. Sci. **31**(2), 122–126 (2019)
3. Ministry of Health, Labour and Welfare of JAPAN: Report on Social Welfare Administration and Services. https://www.mhlw.go.jp/toukei/list/38-1.html (in Japanese)
4. Ministry of Health, Labour and Welfare of JAPAN: Statistics of long-term care benefit expenditures. https://www.mhlw.go.jp/toukei/list/45-1.html (in Japanese)
5. International Organization for Standardization: ISO 7176-8:2014 Wheelchairs Part 8: Requirements and test methods for static, impact and fatigue strengths
6. The Ministry of Health, Labour and Welfare of Japan: Certification Standards and Verification Methods for Seating Support Device Components (Revised Edition 2). https://www.mhlw.go.jp/stf/shingi/2r98520000001hioc-att/2r98520000001hipt.pdf (in Japanese)
7. Shirogane, S., Handa, T., Kozai, Y., Maeda, Y.: A preliminary study of the measurement of overload applied to the foot support of a wheelchair and a seated postural support device. J. Phys. Ther. Sci. **29**(1), 8–11 (2017)
8. Kozai, Y., Sato, H., Handa, T., Suzuki, K., Noto, T., Ando, M., Maeda, Y., Shirogane, S.: Overload on wheelchairs due to spasticity: measurement of forces acting on the head support. Rigakuryoho Kagaku. **33**(1), 49–53 (2018) (in Japanese)
9. Toyama, S., Tanaka, Y., Shirogane, S., Nakamura, T., Umino, T., Uehara, R., Okamoto, T., Igarashi, H.: Development of wearable sheet-type shear force sensor and measurement system: insusceptible to temperature and pressure. Sensors. **17**(8), 1752 (2017)
10. Watanabe, K., Hara, K., Toyama, S.: Development of hybrid three-axis load sensor. Sens. Mater. **32**(2), 779–790 (2020)
11. Shirogane, S., Toyama, S.: Postural hysteresis effect of buttock shear force in wheelchair seating. Jpn. J. Wheelchair Seating. **2**(1), 10–15 (2017) (in Japanese)
12. Shirogane, S., Toyama, S., Takashima, A., Tanaka, T.: The relationship between torso inclination and the shearing force of the buttocks while seated in a wheelchair: preliminary research in non-disabled individuals. Assist. Technol. **32**(6), 287–293 (2020)
13. Shirogane, S., Toyama, S., Hoshino, M., Takashima, A., Tanaka, T.: Quantitative measurement of the pressure and shear stress acting on the body of a wheelchair user using a wearable sheet-type sensor: a preliminary study. Int. J. Environ. Res. Public Health. **19**(20), 13579 (2022)
14. http://www.mhlw.go.jp/stf/houdou/2r9852000002iau1.html
15. Pellichero, A., Kenyon, K.L., Best, L.K., Lamontagne, M.E., Lavoie, D.M., Sorita, E., Routhier, F.: Relationships between cognitive functioning and powered mobility device use: a scoping review. Int. J. Environ. Res. Public Health. **18**(23), 12467 (2021). https://doi.org/10.3390/ijerph182312467
16. Hou, L., Latif, L., Mehryar, P., Withers, S., Plastropoulos, A., Shen, L., Ali, Z.: An autonomous wheelchair with health monitoring system based on internet of thing. Sci. Rep. **14**(1), 5878 (2024). https://doi.org/10.1038/s41598-024-56357-y
17. Tanaka, T., Matsushita, H., Sugihara, S., Izumi, T., Kato, N., Miyasaka, T., Maeda, Y., Nakajima, Y.: Development of new alert system using visual and auditory stimuli to assist patients with cognitive impairment in wheelchair operation. J. Med. Biol. Eng. **35**, 585–593 (2015). https://doi.org/10.1007/s40846-015-0077-9

Chapter 7
Supporting Mobility for the Elderly and Persons with Disabilities 2

Yusuke Maeda and Toshiaki Tanaka

Abstract Section 7.1 introduces welfare engineering research related to gait. Gait rehabilitation using biofeedback has shown high training efficacy for patients with neurological disorders. This method involves measuring biosignals such as Electromyography (EMG) and electroencephalography (EEG) and then using that information to consciously adjust one's own movements. These approaches allow for the noninvasive creation of individualized training content.

Gait training utilizing virtual reality (VR) and robotics makes it possible to set up diverse virtual environments and difficulty levels. In most cases, parameters like walking speed and sway can be quantified, offering advantages not found in conventional gait training. Furthermore, by combining biofeedback with robot-assisted rehabilitation, even higher intervention effects than traditional methods can be expected. In recent years, the development of various devices has enabled training that can intervene in both postural control and cognitive function. For example, dual-task training, such as "thinking while walking," can enhance attention-splitting abilities, leading to improvements in cognitive and physical function, as well as promoting neuroplasticity (the ability to reorganize neural pathways). Artificial intelligence (AI)-powered pose estimation technology allows for low-cost and simple motion capture. As AI learning progresses, its measurement accuracy is also improving dramatically.

This study addresses the growing need for mobility support in aging societies by developing and validating two assistive systems with real-time alert functions. The first system is a personal mobility (PM) system that uses IMU sensors to monitor body posture and detect misalignments between the user and the device. When abnormal joint angle deviations occur, such as between the trunk and backrest,

Y. Maeda
School of Health Sciences at Odawara, International University of Health and Welfare, Kanagawa, Japan
e-mail: y.maeda@ihwg.jp

T. Tanaka (✉)
Research Center for Advanced Science and Technology/Institute of Gerontology, The University of Tokyo, Tokyo, Japan
e-mail: t.tanaka@iog.u-tokyo.ac.jp; tanaka@bfp.rcast.u-tokyo.ac.jp

T. Tanaka (ed.), *Inclusive and Barrier-Free Designs for Rehabilitation Engineering*,
https://doi.org/10.1007/978-981-95-5783-7_7

vibration and voice alerts are triggered. Trials involving healthy adults simulating elderly conditions demonstrated that the alerts were activated within 0.3 s and perceived as effective.

The second system is a walking-assist robot that uses HAL® and curara® exoskeletons. IMU sensors track hip and knee motion; deviations from preset angles trigger haptic alerts. The curara® system further synchronized these alerts with its assistive motions, resulting in smoother, more stable gait patterns. Compared to the HAL® system, the curara® system showed smaller joint deviations and higher user comfort.

Although they are designed for different environments—the PM system for daily mobility and the walking-assist robot system for rehabilitation—both systems share a common architecture involving real-time sensing and multimodal feedback. This study emphasizes the importance of integrating these technologies into a unified support platform that can adapt to the user's context and physical condition.

Future development should combine PM and robotic assistance with AI and the Internet of Things (IoT), enabling personalized, adaptive mobility support that promotes safety and independent living for the elderly and disabled.

7.1 A Review of Assistive Engineering Research on Gait Rehabilitation

7.1.1 Introduction

Walking is a complex movement that involves moving one's entire body while maintaining an upright posture against gravity. It is performed through the coordinated action of the entire musculoskeletal system with the central nervous system working in concert. During bipedal walking, balance is mechanically lost and then regained in a regular and repetitive manner. Sensory systems such as proprioception and the vestibular system are involved in regaining mechanical stability. From a psychological and social perspective, walking is an independent means of mobility that influences social participation and quality of daily life. A decline in walking ability can lead to an increased risk of falls and social isolation, requiring appropriate training and the use of assistive devices. Even older adults, individuals with disabilities, and those with medical conditions can safely move using assistive devices. Furthermore, the appropriate use of assistive devices allows individuals with walking difficulties owing to paralysis or muscle weakness to safely engage in gait training. Improved walking ability expands the range of mobility, facilitates smoother performance in activities of daily living (ADLs), and makes it easier to participate in outings and hobbies, which, in turn, leads to improved quality of life (QOL) and increased motivation for social engagement.

7.1.2 Rehabilitation Using Biofeedback for Patients with Neurological Disorders

Biofeedback has been used in rehabilitation settings for neurological patients such as those with stroke or Parkinson's disease (PD) to facilitate normal movement patterns after neurological injury. Cha et al. reported that gait training with auditory feedback regarding heel-loading sensations in stroke hemiplegic patients resulted in improved gait and balance outcomes [1]. A study involving patients with PD who underwent 8 weeks of treadmill gait training with vibration stimulation applied to the soles of their feet showed improvements in gait speed, stride length, and lower limb joint range of motion (ROM). Crea et al. reported on biofeedback therapy for individuals with transfemoral prostheses [2]. They conducted training on a treadmill equipped with a feedback device that controlled a vibrotactile stimulation unit based on signals from sensorized insoles along with visual feedback regarding the temporal symmetry of gait. This temporarily improved gait symmetry. Electroencephalography (EEG) and EMG detect and record signals from the brain and muscles. Regarding EEG use, results have indicated that improvements in the performance of patients with PD can be achieved by activating specific brain regions such as the central parietal to parietal central (CPz-PCz) through video games and other means before training [3]. The use of EMG has been primarily reported with sensors placed on the gastrocnemius and tibialis anterior muscles, often combined with visual or auditory feedback to activate these muscles [4, 5].

7.1.3 VR-Based Gait Rehabilitation

VR has been employed in motor therapy for PD, stroke, and other neurological disorders. In walking-in-place interfaces, users make stepping-like movements without physically moving forward; instead, a virtual forward movement is induced [6]. This allows for the acquisition of proprioceptive feedback similar to actual walking [7]. Redirected walking causes users to have different perceptions when walking in the virtual world compared to the real world. This makes it possible to significantly reduce the space required for gait training. There are reports that dual-task loading with cognitive tasks during step training in patients with PD reduces the number of freezing of gait episodes [8]. Furthermore, VR enhances and manipulates visual information, suggesting its potential to modify gait characteristics in patients with PD or stroke [9, 10].

7.1.4 Robot-Assisted Gait and Balance Training

Various modalities are available, including robot-assisted training with mechanical electrical stimulation, ankle robots, end-effector devices, and seated rehabilitation robots. Robotic devices can provide "repetitive task training." Furthermore, they eliminate the need for therapists to manually position paralyzed limbs or assist with trunk movements, thereby reducing the physical burden on therapists [11]. The results indicated that patients with stroke who underwent robot-assisted gait training were more likely to achieve independent walking than those who received conventional gait training alone [12]. Because walking speed during robot-assisted gait training is faster than that during conventional gait training, patients can repeat a greater number of gait cycles [13].

7.1.5 Gait Training Using Exoskeletons

Regarding research using exoskeletons, a previous study evaluated patients with stroke who underwent 6–8 weeks of training using a smart medical actuator (SMA). Although both the functional task-specific training (FTST) group and SMA groups showed improvements in walking ability, the SMA group demonstrated improvements in a greater number of gait parameters [14]. Watanabe et al. compared the effectiveness of gait training using a unilateral version of the Hybrid Assistive Limb® to that of conventional gait training in patients in the chronic phase of stroke recovery. Compared to the conventional group, the Hybrid Assistive Limb® group showed significant improvement in the functional ambulation categories after 12 sessions following 4 weeks of training, as well as at 8-week and 12-week follow-ups [15]. Calabro et al. compared robot-assisted training using Ekso combined with conventional gait training with conventional gait training alone. The robotic group demonstrated significant improvements in walking speed, corticospinal excitability, and muscle activation [16].

7.1.6 Gait Assessment Via Low-Invasive Methods

Following recent trends in telehealth, healthcare support and management are increasingly shifting from hospital to home settings. Radiofrequency technology enables the easier and more precise tracking of patient movements. These offer advantages, such as low power consumption, no need for attachment, low noise, and high temporal resolution, with fewer privacy concerns. The combination of ultra-wideband (UWB) and inertial measurement unit (IMU) has improved the accuracy of patient localization in home settings [17]. A low-cost and less complex wireless gait tracking system suitable for both indoor and outdoor measurements using wearable UWB transceivers was devised. The proposed system could detect the distance from the knee to the foot with high accuracy [18]. A wearable system based on a pair of small, lightweight UWB antennas placed near the heel and toe of the foot can measure gait clearance [19]. Mastorakis and Makris designed a fall detection model that recognizes when the height, width, and depth of a 3D bounding box enclosing a human silhouette exceed certain thresholds [20]. Zhang and Liu detected falls using a depth reference image to detect the head region from the human body and floor plane [21].

7.1.7 Gait Analysis Using a Brain-Computer Interface (BCI)

EEG and functional near-infrared spectroscopy (fNIRS) are among the most commonly used techniques for monitoring brain activity because of their portability, noninvasiveness, and relatively low cost compared with other technologies. EEG-based robot-assisted gait rehabilitation has the potential to improve mobility in patients with stroke [8]. By utilizing EEG-based neural decoding, it is possible to develop patient-specific closed-loop EEG-BCI systems that can enhance lower limb rehabilitation and encourage cortical plasticity [22]. The combination of EEG and fNIRS helps to detect changes in the spatial and temporal information of cortical activation patterns, contributing to a better understanding of robot-assisted gait rehabilitation [23].

7.1.8 Dual-Task Gait Training Utilizing Assistive Devices

The use of innovative technology interfaces allows participants to perform motor and cognitive activities simultaneously during cognitive-motor dual-task training (CMDT). CMDT refers to the concurrent processing of motor (e.g., walking, gait initiation, balance, and physical movement) and cognitive (e.g., attention, decision-making, and working memory) activities. Such interactions between cognitive and motor abilities are observed in cognitive functions, such as attention and executive functions, and motor activities, such as gait, balance, and motor control. However, when the demand for performing two tasks simultaneously exceeds cognitive-motor skills, the performance of one or both tasks may be affected [24]. CMDT may be beneficial, considering its effects on frontal lobe cognitive and motor functions [25, 26]. Several studies have reported technology-assisted CMDT in older adults. Fifty-six older adults with mild to moderate dementia participated in a 10-week training program, twice a week, using an exergaming-based balance training system (Physiomat®) that combined postural control tasks with a cognitive task from a neuropsychological test (Trail Making Test). The training resulted in a significant reduction in completion time [27]. There have been reports on the effectiveness of a CMDT program using a semi-immersive dual-task virtual room featuring three haptic carpets (smooth, sandy, and cobblestone), a video projector, five screens, a walkable LED floor, and audio [28]. They concluded that cognitive-motor exercises such as associating sounds and images with memory, walking while searching for numbers, and performing calculations are effective methods for improving gait stability, gait patterns, walking speed, and fear of falling. Twenty patients with PD underwent 18 sessions (3 times per week) of progressive focused treadmill training using VR obstacles [29]. Significant improvements were observed in the walking speed during normal walking, dual-tasking, and stepping over ground obstacles. Furthermore, variability in dual-task walking decreased (improved), and trail-making test times also improved. Additionally, enhanced functional performance measures and retention effects were observed 1 month later. This indicates the potential to significantly improve physical abilities, walking in complex and challenging situations, and specific aspects of cognitive function in patients with PD. Mirelman et al. randomly assigned 302 adults aged 60–90 years at high risk for falling, who had various motor and cognitive impairments, to either a 6-week treadmill training program combined with VR or a treadmill training program alone and then compared the training effects between the groups [30]. The VR system consisted of motion capture cameras and a computer-generated simulation projected onto a large screen specifically designed to reduce the fall risk in older adults by incorporating real-world challenges such as obstacles, multiple pathways, and distractors requiring continuous step adjustments. The VR-combined group showed a significantly greater reduction in fall rate compared to the treadmill-only group.

7.1.9 Gait Analysis Using Other Diverse Devices and Sensors

EMG is a technique that records and measures muscle activity, with surface EMG being particularly utilized in research on gait event extraction, phase recognition of normal and pathological gaits, and muscle fatigue. Chorin et al. analyzed EMG and force data from 40 subjects (10 elderly fallers and 30 non-fallers) and found a significant difference in lateral gastrocnemius muscle activity between the faller and non-faller groups [31]. Fujita et al. measured lower limb EMG during prolonged walking in patients with stroke-induced hemiplegia and reported that the mean instantaneous frequency significantly decreased in the non-paretic tibialis anterior and paretic rectus femoris, showing a waveform pattern different from that of healthy individuals [32]. Force myography (FMG) measures the pressure exerted by the muscles during activity. When wrapped around a relevant area using a bracelet or socket, the sensors can measure the outward force generated by the volume changes resulting from the displacement of the muscles, tendons, and skin. Lukowicz et al. reported that signal patterns from force-sensitive resistors worn on the thigh could distinguish between four types of gait [33]. Yungher et al. demonstrated a correlation between FMG (surface muscle pressure) and surface muscle electrical activity during walking [34], noting that FMG signal patterns exhibited greater stride-to-stride consistency than surface electromyography (sEMG) signals. Similarly, Belyea et al. corroborated the correlation between FMG and sEMG signals and identified FMG signals as potentially better indicators of fatigue levels [35]. Piezoelectric sensors generate an electrical potential when subjected to mechanical stress and are commonly used to measure dynamic pressure and vibration. They can be used for triaxial measurements, which allows them to generate positive or negative (amplitude) electrical impulses depending on the direction of the force acting around each axis [36]. Gait recognition technology using flexible piezoelectric sensors [polyvinylidene fluoride (PVDF)] was reported by Cha et al. Four sensors, one attached to each knee and hip on both sides, generated a voltage corresponding to the flexion of the respective limb joints. The periodic motion components extracted from the Fast Fourier Transform (FFT) of the signals changing over time were correlated with the walking speed. This system can detect postural changes during standing and walking [1]. Using a wearable microphone to record the interaction between the foot and ground during walking (footsteps) can reveal important aspects of gait. Microphone sensors are highly practical for capturing footsteps generated by the impact of the foot on the ground because of their small size, low cost, portability, and ease of integration with embedded electronics. Wang et al. attempted to record gait events using wearable microphones [37]. Microphones attached to both feet were used to collect sounds originating from different parts of the foot. Based on spectral analysis of the sounds, a set of 36 features was extracted, including correlation coefficients, energy bands, zero-crossing rate, linear prediction, and mel-frequency cepstral coefficients. A support vector machine (SVM)-based approach was used to identify and classify step detection, initial contact, and toe off, and sound data from both feet were fused to estimate nine spatiotemporal parameter sets. Jesus et al. published a case report estimating the gait rhythm, velocity, and step/stride duration in a patient (stage 3 on the Hoehn and Yahr scale) using gait acoustic signals captured using a microphone [38]. Cases describing the use of ear-worn wearable (earable) microphones for gait identification have been reported. Ferlini et al. used the EarGate system that employs inward-facing earphones to leverage the occlusion effect (low-frequency components of bone-conducted sounds when the ear canal opening is sealed) while the wearer is moving. According to this study, 31 healthy subjects were identified with an accuracy >97% [39]. Ultrasonic sensors calculate the distance to an object by emitting short high-frequency sound waves at regular intervals. Recent ultrasonic sensors can measure minute changes in distance, suggesting their potential for use in gait analysis applications. An ultrasonic transmitter fixed at an arbitrary indoor location sent periodic bursts of pulses to two receivers attached to the subject's feet. The propagation delay recorded between transmission and reception allows for the localization of the subject's feet. Information regarding foot position and instances of zero foot velocity can be used to calculate the step and stride lengths [40]. Another study by Qi et al. reported the use of a wireless ultrasonic sensor network to measure foot trajectories in 3D [41].

7.1.10 Gait Analysis Using OpenCap (Pose Estimation Artificial Intelligence [AI])

Although devices such as three-dimensional motion capture systems and video analysis are highly useful and well-established methodologies for gait analysis, they also have drawbacks. These include high costs, which can hinder their adoption, and the time-consuming process of attaching markers, leading to a significant burden on subjects. Therefore, in recent years, methods using AI for pose estimation have garnered attention as affordable and convenient tools for gait analysis. OpenCap, which is capable of capturing motion with just two smartphones, facilitates measurements not only in laboratory settings but also in clinical environments and outdoors. Furthermore, because it eliminates the need for reflective marker placement, the burden on subjects is minimal. Uhlrich et al. [42] reported that the use of OpenCap resulted in costs of $<1\%$ compared to laboratory-based measurement and analysis, with a significantly faster processing time. Kanko et al. validated the accuracy of pose estimation AI in gait analysis by combining conventional motion capture systems with markerless motion capture. Their findings indicated a high similarity in the estimated values for the lower limb joint angles and joint center positions between markerless and marker-based motion capture, highlighting the practical utility of AI-driven pose estimation. This is supported by the findings in [43, 44]. According to Needham et al. [45], the analysis of sprinting movements using OpenPose, in conjunction with signal processing techniques such as filtering, has shown promise in estimating Center of Mass (COM) to a certain extent. However, COM estimation can have larger errors for movements other than walking, and its ability to fully capture complex motions is limited.

7.2 Integrated Alert System for Mobility Support: Merging Personal Mobility and Robot-Assisted Technologies

7.2.1 Introduction

With Japan's rapidly aging society, the importance of mobility support technologies is growing. Providing safe and efficient mobility is especially essential for elderly individuals and those with physical limitations to maintain their quality of life (QOL). Until now, assistive devices such as walkers and powered wheelchairs have been widely used. However, due to recent advancements in robotics technology, more advanced support devices have emerged, including walking-assist robots and personal mobility (PM) systems.

In Western countries, lightweight, highly flexible assistive devices that incorporate soft robotics have been developed to complement physical function and stabilize gait in the elderly. For instance, Tricomi et al. found that soft robotic shorts called "WalkON," which assist with hip flexion, significantly reduce the metabolic cost of

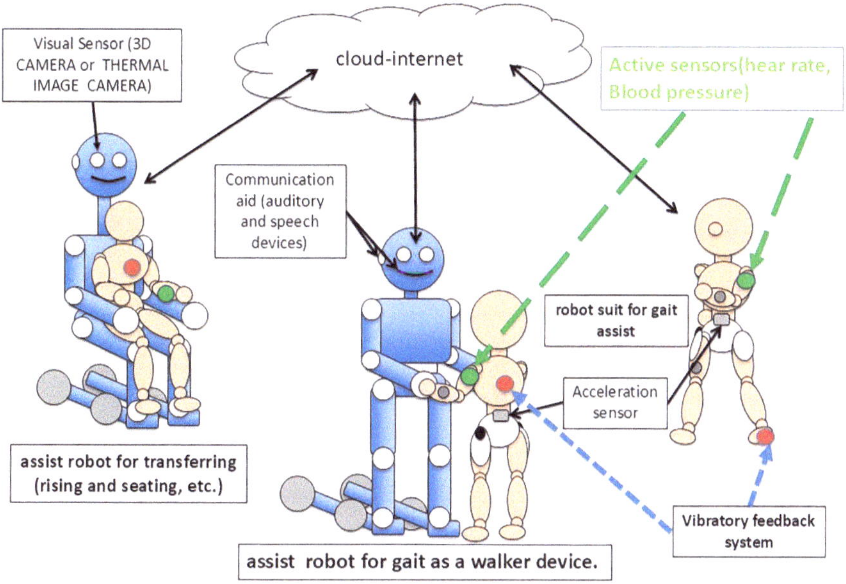

Fig. 7.1 A total assist robot for gait and transferring and communication

walking and enable older adults to walk long distances [46]. Additionally, Morris et al. noted the rigidity issues of conventional exoskeleton-type robots and suggested that introducing more adaptable soft robotic systems could achieve safety and comfort simultaneously [47]. In Japan, the application of walking-assist robots, such as HAL®, in clinical rehabilitation is also being actively pursued [48].

Based on these domestic and international trends, the present study aims to promote the independence of the elderly and prevent falls by developing mobility support systems with alert functions. Specifically, the system uses inertial measurement unit (IMU) sensors to synchronously measure the user's body movement and the device's motion. This allows the system to detect abnormal movements and posture changes in real time and provide visual, auditory, and tactile feedback. This "alert system" is the core of the proposed technology (Figs. 7.1 and 7.2).

7.2.2 Development of a Personal Mobility System with Alert Function

7.2.2.1 Objective

The objective of this section is to develop a new type of assistive device that integrates an alert system into a personal mobility (PM) platform. Traditional PM systems mainly focus on providing transportation and lack dynamic feedback

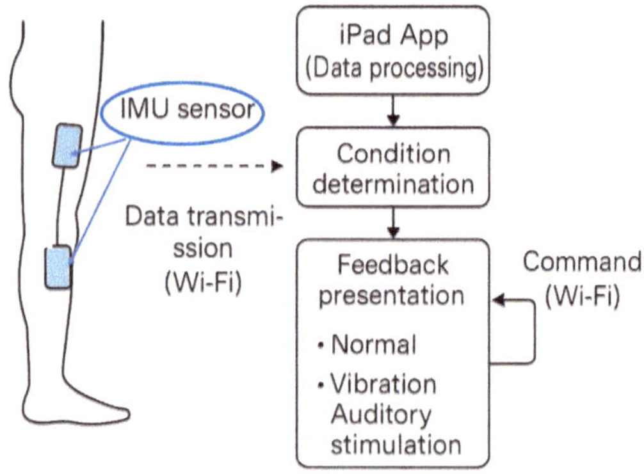

Fig. 7.2 IMU based alert system for supporting gait with the PM and the assist robot

functions that synchronize with the user's body. This study aims to create a system that monitors joint movement in real time. When hazardous posture changes are detected, the system provides immediate voice guidance and vibration alerts.

7.2.2.2 Method

Five healthy adult males in their 20s participated in the experiment. Wearing elderly-simulation gear, such as weighted vests and vision/hearing restriction equipment, they operated a Permobil F5 powered wheelchair®. The participants performed everyday transfer movements, such as "sitting to supine" and "supine to standing." IMU sensors were attached to the users' trunks, hips, knees, and ankles, and the same types of sensors were placed on the corresponding parts of the wheelchair. The system was designed to issue 100Hz vibration stimulation and voice guidance to prompt postural correction when the deviation in joint angle exceeded a preset threshold in Figs. 7.3, 7.4, and 7.5 [49].

7.2.2.3 Results

The experimental results showed that the average deviation in angle between the trunk and the backrest was 18.7°, with a maximum deviation of 24°. Deviations of approximately 10–20° were also observed between the hip and seat, knee and leg support, and ankle and footrest. When these deviations exceeded the threshold, alerts were triggered within an average of 0.3 s, and all participants perceived the feedback. Subjective evaluations also indicated that the system effectively suppressed unintended or incorrect posture.

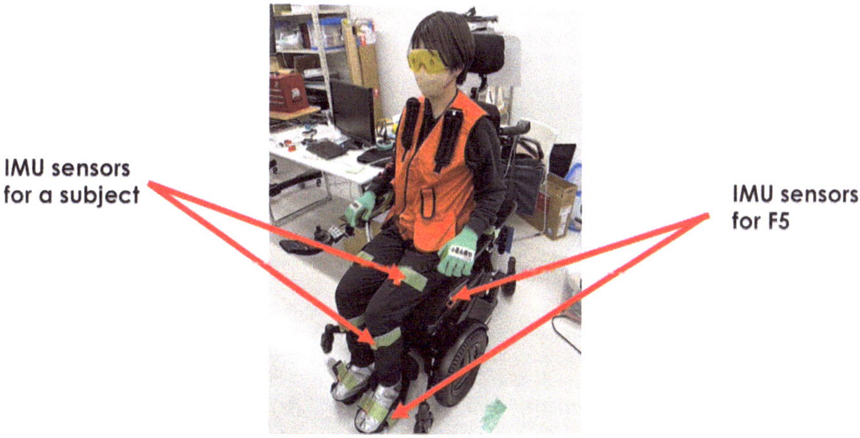

Fig. 7.3 Sitting position of a subject in a F5 wheelchair wearing the elderly experience simulation

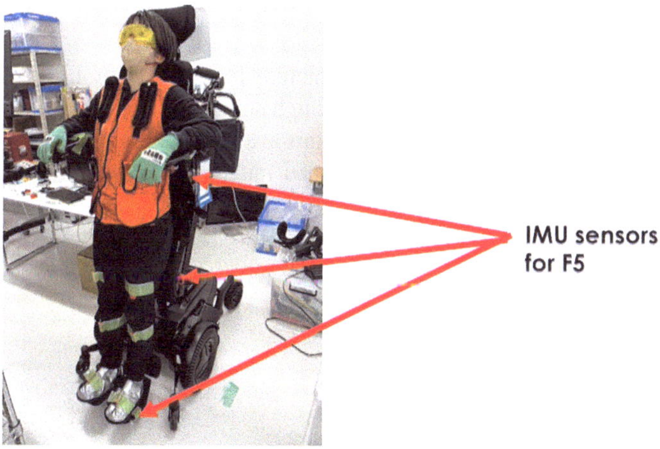

Fig. 7.4 Standing position of a subject in a F5 wheelchair wearing the elderly experience simulation

7.2.3 Development of a Walking-Assist Robot with an Alert System

7.2.3.1 Objective

The objective of this section is to enhance walking safety during rehabilitation and daily life by integrating an alert system into a walking-assist robot. This system is specifically intended for elderly individuals and poststroke patients who need to relearn motor functions. This study verifies the effectiveness of a system that issues real-time warnings when abnormal joint motion occurs while walking.

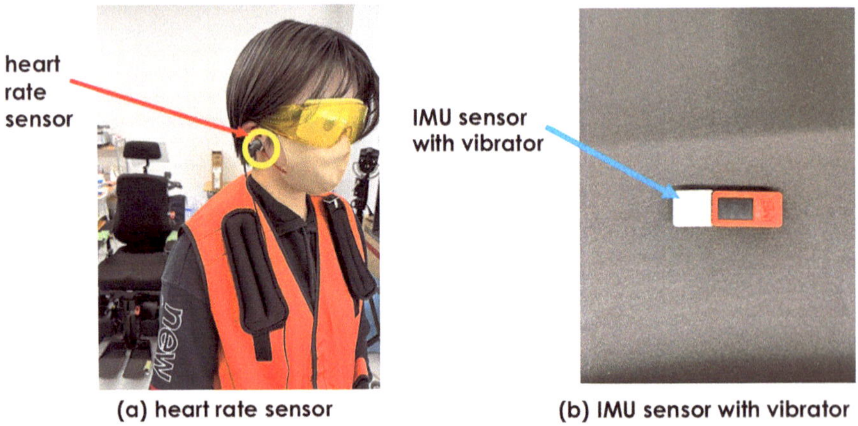

Fig. 7.5 New alert system for vibration and heart rate devices

7.2.3.2 Method

Walking-assist devices used in this study included the exoskeleton-type HAL® and curara®. IMU sensors were attached to the thigh and lower leg to measure the flexion and extension angles of the hip and knee joints at a sampling rate of 10 Hz. When the joint angles deviated from the predetermined range during walking, the vibration module, which was mounted on the thigh, was activated to alert the user through haptic stimulation. Additionally, Figs. 7.6 and 7.7 [50] show the investigation of synchronized control of the vibration stimulation with the walking assistance pattern for the curara® system.

7.2.3.3 Results (Table 7.1)

When using the HAL®, the maximum angular deviation observed was 23.7° at the hip joint and 9.9° at the knee joint. With curara®, the respective deviations were 16.5° and 3.6°. The curara® system exhibited high synchronization between vibration feedback and motion control patterns, enabling alerts to be issued without disrupting walking continuity. Participants reported that they could perceive the warnings without discomfort, suggesting that the system strikes a balance between safety and usability.

7.2.4 Discussion

The two systems developed in this study—a personal mobility (PM)-based system and a walking-assist-type mobility support device with integrated alert

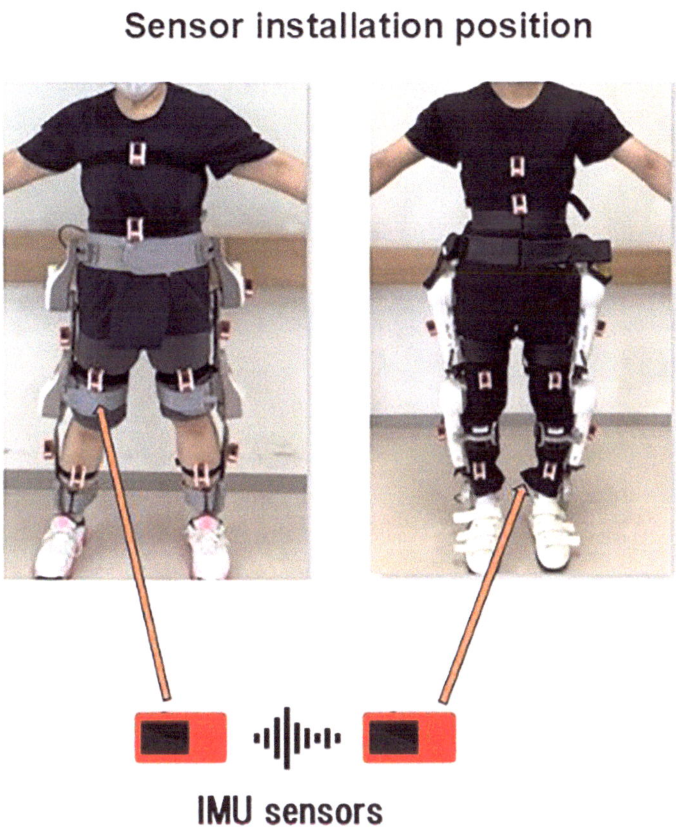

Fig. 7.6 IMU sensor installation on assist robot and human body

functionality—are designed for different usage environments, yet they share a common foundation in real-time sensing and feedback mechanisms. The PM system contributes to mobility support both indoors and outdoors, while the walking-assist robot enhances gait safety during rehabilitation and daily activities.

Western research has reported on the long-term effectiveness of gait assistance using soft robotics. According to a study by Jin et al., 6 weeks of continuous use improved gait speed and stability. Gait symmetry improved by an average of 9.8% [51]. Furthermore, the flexible exoskeleton design reduced wearers' fatigue and improved their endurance during physical activity.

Based on these findings, future development should aim to create a "hybrid-type mobility support device" that integrates both PM and walking-assist functionalities (Fig. 7.1). Designing systems that allow users to switch assistance modes flexibly according to the situation is necessary to select the appropriate type of support. Furthermore, a key future challenge is constructing an adaptive alert system that

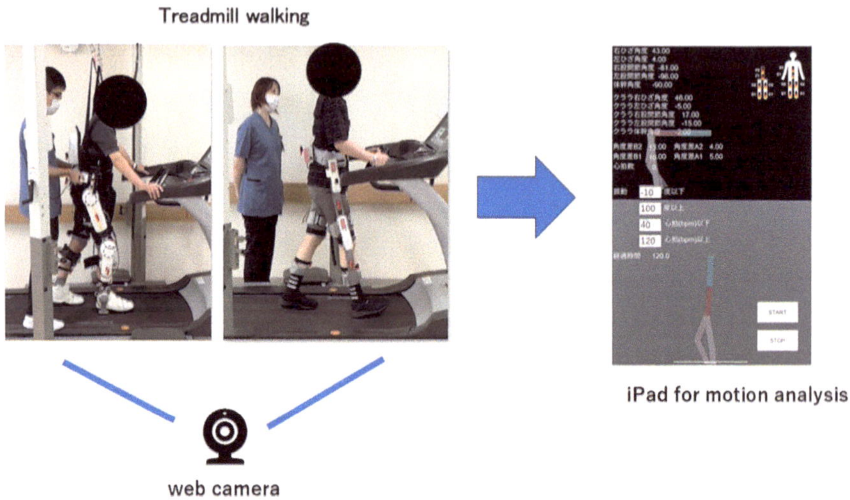

Fig. 7.7 IMU data collection during treadmill walking with assist robot

Table 7.1 Mean joint angle differences per gait cycle between subject and robot systems (HAL® and curara ®)

HAL ©		curara ©	
Hip joint	Knee joint	Hip joint	Knee joint
23.7 ± 8.5°	9.9 ± 8.3°	16.5 ± 6.7°	3.6 ± 6.5°

analyzes sensor data through AI to deliver optimized, real-time assistance tailored to each user.

7.2.5 Conclusion

This study developed two mobility assistance devices, one based on personal mobility (PM) and the other on a walking-assist robot, both with integrated alert systems. Their respective effectiveness was experimentally validated. Using IMU sensors to measure joint angles and provide real-time feedback demonstrated that discrepancies between user movement and device motion could be detected and immediately alerted.

While each device can function independently to provide effective support, future efforts should focus on integrating them to create a "unified alert-equipped mobility assistance system" that responds to users' living environments and physical conditions. Linking such systems with AI, IoT, and cloud technologies in the future will allow for more personalized support and the realization of a society that fosters independence.

References

1. Cha, Y., Kim, H., Kim, D.: Flexible piezoelectric sensor-based gait recognition. Sensors. **18**(2), 468 (2018)
2. Crea, S., et al.: Time-discrete vibrotactile feedback contributes to improved gait symmetry in patients with lower limb amputations: case series. Phys. Ther. **97**(2), 198–207 (2017)
3. Azarpaikan, A., Torbati, H.T., Sohrabi, M.: Neurofeedback and physical balance in Parkinson's patients. Gait Posture. **40**(1), 177–181 (2014)
4. Intiso, D., et al.: Rehabilitation of walking with electromyographic biofeedback in foot-drop after stroke. Stroke. **25**(6), 1189–1192 (1994)
5. Mandel, A.R., et al.: Electromyographic versus rhythmic positional biofeedback in computerized gait retraining with stroke patients. Arch. Phys. Med. Rehabil. **71**(9), 649–654 (1990)
6. Janeh, O., Steinicke, F.: A review of the potential of virtual walking techniques for gait rehabilitation. Front. Hum. Neurosci. **15**, 717291 (2021)
7. Slater, M., Usoh, M., Steed, A.: Steps and ladders in virtual reality. In: Virtual Reality Software and Technology, pp. 45–54
8. Killane, I., et al.: Dual motor-cognitive virtual reality training impacts dual-task performance in freezing of gait. IEEE J. Biomed. Health Inform. (2015)
9. Lamontagne, A., et al.: Modulation of walking speed by changing optic flow in persons with stroke. J. Neuroeng. Rehabil. **4**, 22 (2007)
10. Schubert, M., et al.: Visual kinesthesia and locomotion in Parkinson's disease. Mov. Disord. **20**(2), 141–150 (2005)
11. Esquenazi, A., Packel, A.: Robotic-assisted gait training and restoration. Am. J. Phys. Med. Rehabil. **91**(11), S217–S231 (2012)
12. Mehrholz, J., et al.: Electromechanical-assisted training for walking after stroke. Cochrane Database Syst. Rev. **5**(5), Cd006185 (2017)
13. van Nunen, M.P., et al.: Exercise intensity of robot-assisted walking versus overground walking in nonambulatory stroke patients. J. Rehabil. Res. Dev. **49**(10), 1537–1546 (2012)
14. Buesing, C., et al.: Effects of a wearable exoskeleton stride management assist system (SMA®) on spatiotemporal gait characteristics in individuals after stroke: a randomized controlled trial. J. Neuroeng. Rehabil. **12**(1), 69 (2015)
15. Watanabe, H., et al.: Effects of gait training using the hybrid assistive limb® in recovery-phase stroke patients: a 2-month follow-up, randomized, controlled study. NeuroRehabilitation. **40**(3), 363–367 (2017)
16. Calabrò, R.S., et al.: Shaping neuroplasticity by using powered exoskeletons in patients with stroke: a randomized clinical trial. J. Neuroeng. Rehabil. **15**(1), 35 (2018)
17. Wang, Y., Li, X.: The IMU/UWB fusion positioning algorithm based on a particle filter. ISPRS Int. J. Geo Inf. **6**(8), 235 (2017)
18. Shaban, H.A., El-Nasr, M.A., Buehrer, R.M.: Toward a highly accurate ambulatory system for clinical gait analysis via UWB radios. IEEE Trans. Inf. Technol. Biomed. **14**(2), 284–291 (2010)
19. Qi, Y., et al.: Using wearable UWB radios to measure foot clearance during walking. Annu. Int. Conf. IEEE Eng. Med. Biol. Soc. **2013**, 5199–5202 (2013)
20. Mastorakis, G., Makris, D.: Fall detection system using Kinect's infrared sensor. J. Real-Time Image Proc. **9**(4), 635–646 (2014)
21. Zhang, Z., et al.: A viewpoint-independent statistical method for fall detection. In: Proceedings of the 21st International Conference on Pattern Recognition (ICPR2012) (2012)
22. Contreras-Vidal, J.L., et al.: Neural decoding of robot-assisted gait during rehabilitation after stroke. Am. J. Phys. Med. Rehabil. **97**(8), 541–550 (2018)
23. Berger, A., et al.: Current state and future prospects of EEG and fNIRS in robot-assisted gait rehabilitation: a brief review. Front. Hum. Neurosci. **13**, 172 (2019)

24. Bayot, M., et al.: The interaction between cognition and motor control: a theoretical framework for dual-task interference effects on posture, gait initiation, gait and turning. Neurophysiol. Clin. **48**(6), 361–375 (2018)
25. Calderón-Larrañaga, A., et al.: Assessing and measuring chronic multimorbidity in the older population: a proposal for its operationalization. J. Gerontol. A Biol. Sci. Med. Sci. **72**(10), 1417–1423 (2017)
26. Kahya, M., et al.: Brain activity during dual task gait and balance in aging and age-related neurodegenerative conditions: a systematic review. Exp. Gerontol. **128**, 110756 (2019)
27. Werner, C., et al.: Time course of changes in motor-cognitive exergame performances during task-specific training in patients with dementia: identification and predictors of early training response. J. Neuroeng. Rehabil. **15**(1), 100 (2018)
28. Spanò, B., et al.: Effect of dual-task motor-cognitive training in preventing falls in vulnerable elderly cerebrovascular patients: a pilot study. Brain Sci. **12**(2) (2022)
29. Mirelman, A., et al.: Virtual reality for gait training: can it induce motor learning to enhance complex walking and reduce fall risk in patients with Parkinson's disease? J. Gerontol. A. **66A**(2), 234–240 (2010)
30. Mirelman, A., et al.: Addition of a non-immersive virtual reality component to treadmill training to reduce fall risk in older adults (V-TIME): a randomised controlled trial. Lancet. **388**(10050), 1170–1182 (2016)
31. Chorin, F., et al.: Sit to stand in elderly fallers vs non-fallers: new insights from force platform and electromyography data. Aging Clin. Exp. Res. **28**(5), 871–879 (2016)
32. Fujita, K., Kobayashi, Y., Hitosugi, M.: Temporal changes in electromyographic activity and gait ability during extended walking in individuals post-stroke: a pilot study. Healthcare (Basel). **9**(4) (2021)
33. Lukowicz, P., et al.: Detecting and interpreting muscle activity with wearable force sensors. In: Pervasive Computing. Springer Berlin Heidelberg, Berlin, Heidelberg (2006)
34. Yungher, D.A., et al.: Surface muscle pressure as a measure of active and passive behavior of muscles during gait. Med. Eng. Phys. **33**(4), 464–471 (2011)
35. Belyea, A.T., Englehart, K.B., Scheme, E.J.: A proportional control scheme for high density force myography. J. Neural Eng. **15**(4), 046029 (2018)
36. Das, R., et al.: Recent trends and practices toward assessment and rehabilitation of neurodegenerative disorders: insights from human gait. Front. Neurosci. **16**, 859298 (2022)
37. Wang, C., et al.: Estimation of temporal gait parameters using a wearable microphone-sensor-based system. Sensors (Basel). **16**(12) (2016)
38. Jesus, J., et al., A microphone-based gait assessment method (MGAM) in a patient with Parkinson disease. A case report. 2019: p. 25-33
39. Ferlini, A., et al.: EarGate: gait-based user identification with in-ear microphones. In: Proceedings of the 27th Annual International Conference on Mobile Computing and Networking, pp. 337–349. Association for Computing Machinery, New Orleans (2021)
40. Huitema, R.B., Hof, A.L., Postema, K.: Ultrasonic motion analysis system—measurement of temporal and spatial gait parameters. J. Biomech. **35**(6), 837–842 (2002)
41. Qi, Y., et al.: Ambulatory measurement of three-dimensional foot displacement during treadmill walking using wearable wireless ultrasonic sensor network. IEEE J. Biomed. Health Inform. **19**(2), 446–452 (2015)
42. Uhlrich, S.D., et al.: OpenCap: 3D human movement dynamics from smartphone videos. bioRxiv. p. 2022.07.07.499061 (2022)
43. Kanko, R.M., et al.: Inter-session repeatability of markerless motion capture gait kinematics. J. Biomech. **121**, 110422 (2021)
44. Kanko, R.M., et al.: Concurrent assessment of gait kinematics using marker-based and markerless motion capture. J. Biomech. **127**, 110665 (2021)
45. Needham, L., et al.: Can markerless pose estimation algorithms estimate 3D mass Centre positions and velocities during linear sprinting activities? Sensors (Basel). **21**(8) (2021)

46. Tricomi, E., Missiroli, F., Xiloyannis, M., et al.: Soft robotic shorts improve outdoor walking efficiency in older adults. In: Nature Machine Intelligence, vol. 6, pp. 1145–1155. Nature Publishing Group (2024). https://doi.org/10.1038/s42256-024-00894-8
47. Morris, L., Diteesawat, R.S., Rahman, N., et al.: The state-of-the-art of soft robotics to assist mobility: a review of physiotherapist and patient identified limitations of current lower-limb exoskeletons and the potential soft-robotic solutions. J. Neuroeng. Rehabil. **20**, Article 18 (2023) BioMed Central
48. Sankai, Y., Sakurai, T.: Clinical applications of HAL (Hybrid Assistive Limb) for neuromuscular rehabilitation in Japan. Adv. Robot. **32**(11), 585–592. Taylor & Francis (2018). https://doi.org/10.1080/01691864.2018.1452610
49. Tanaka, T., Miura, T.: Effects of postural control by personal mobility on human joint movements—prototype of a new alert system. Ann. Musculoskelet. Med. **8**(1), 001–005. Organ Science Group (2024). https://doi.org/10.17352/amm.000034
50. Tanaka, T., Matsumura, R., Miura, T.: Influence of varied load assistance with exoskeleton-type robotic device on gait rehabilitation. Int. J. Environ. Res. Public Health. **19**(15), 9713. MDPI (2022). https://doi.org/10.3390/ijerph19159713
51. Jin, S., Xiong, X., Zhao, D., Jin, C., Yamamoto, M.: Long-term effects of a soft robotic suit on gait characteristics in healthy elderly persons. Sci. Rep. **13**(1), 32335. Nature Publishing Group (2023). https://doi.org/10.1038/s41598-023-32335-8

Chapter 8
Support at Home and in the Community

Yasuhiro Nakajima, Rika Miura, Naomi Esashi, Shujirou Imaeda, Toshio Otsuki, and Toshiaki Tanaka

Abstract As Japan's population ages, the demand for home-based rehabilitation is growing, particularly in rural areas where resources are limited. This study examines the clinical effectiveness and feasibility of a telerehabilitation system that uses virtual reality (VR) and multisensory feedback. The system uses visual, auditory, and vibratory stimuli to help people with stroke or age-related motor impairments recover motor function.

Three previously developed systems were combined and evaluated through clinical trials involving elderly individuals and people with disabilities. Improvements in joint mobility, movement speed, and balance were observed and supported by clinical assessments and 3D motion analysis. Communication tools such as Skype® and PubNub® enabled effective real-time interaction, confirming the system's suitability for home use.

This study underscores the potential of low-cost information and communications technology (ICT)-based systems to enhance motor learning and daily functioning.

Y. Nakajima (✉)
Human Technology Research Division, Industrial Research Institute, Industrial Technology and Environment Research Department, Local Independent Administrative Agency, Hokkaido Research Organization, Hokkaido, Japan
e-mail: nakajima-yasuhiro@hro.or.jp

R. Miura · N. Esashi
Non-Profit Organization Piskari, Tokyo, Japan

S. Imaeda
Urban Development and Planning Department, Nikken Sekkei Research Institute, Tokyo, Japan
e-mail: imaeda.shujiro@nikken.jp

T. Otsuki
Department of Architecture, Graduate School of Engineering, The University of Tokyo, Tokyo, Japan
e-mail: bigmoon@arch.t.u-tokyo.ac.jp

T. Tanaka (✉)
Research Center for Advanced Science and Technology/Institute of Gerontology, The University of Tokyo, Tokyo, Japan
e-mail: t.tanaka@iog.u-tokyo.ac.jp; tanaka@bfp.rcast.u-tokyo.ac.jp

T. Tanaka (ed.), *Inclusive and Barrier-Free Designs for Rehabilitation Engineering*,
https://doi.org/10.1007/978-981-95-5783-7_8

While promising, challenges remain in simplifying user interfaces and assessing long-term impact. Future developments aim to incorporate AI and the Internet of Things (IoT), but broader support is needed for widespread adoption.

This study examined the effectiveness of a newly developed wedge-type support device for posture retention during therapeutic horseback riding among older adults. Experiments were conducted with both skilled and unskilled riders. Skilled riders were generally able to maintain an appropriate posture even without the device, but their stability further improved when the support was applied. In contrast, unskilled riders initially showed notable postural deviations, but with the use of support, clear improvements in the alignment of the neck, trunk, and lower limbs were observed. In addition, qualitative evaluations revealed favorable ratings for both skilled and unskilled riders, with particularly remarkable improvements in the unskilled group. The usability assessment indicated high overall satisfaction, with skilled riders tending to prefer supports with smaller tilt angles, whereas unskilled riders favored those with greater tilt. These results suggest that the wedge-type support device has the potential to enhance both safety and effectiveness of horseback riding therapy in older adults.

The Hokkaido Industrial Research Institute has developed an S-shaped snow shovel to reduce the physical burden of manual snow removal. Through motion analysis and muscle fatigue measurements, the bent-handle shovel was shown to improve posture and reduce muscular strain. Furthermore, usability evaluations demonstrated higher ratings compared to the traditional straight-handle shovel. Based on these findings, the S-handle shovel has been commercialized and is currently available on the market.

Falls among the older adults are a leading cause of injury, disability, and loss of independence, with a particularly high incidence occurring in the home. This paper examines the role of barrier-free housing design in fall prevention through a comparative analysis of Japanese and international policies, an investigation of architectural risk factors within residences, and a case study of fall circumstances based on home visit surveys conducted by the Institute of Gerontology (IOG) at the University of Tokyo. It also introduces an augmented reality (AR) application developed collaboratively by researchers from the University of Tokyo, Osaka University, the National Institute of Advanced Industrial Science and Technology (AIST), and the Nikken Sekkei Research Institute to visualize fall risks. Finally, the paper discusses future directions for interdisciplinary collaboration among architecture, welfare, medicine, and information technology.

8.1 A Study on Telerehabilitation Systems

8.1.1 Introduction

Japan is one of the world's leading super-aged societies. It is projected that by 2025, approximately 30% of the total population will be 65 years of age or older [1]. As the population ages, the number of individuals suffering from stroke or age-related motor impairments is increasing rapidly. This heightens the need for continued rehabilitation at home [2]. However, human and temporal resources for home visits are limited, particularly in rural and depopulated areas, where it is difficult to provide adequate services [3].

Against this backdrop, telerehabilitation technology is garnering attention. It involves using information and communications technology (ICT) to enable physical and occupational therapists to remotely provide exercise guidance and feedback to patients. This system provides continuous, high-quality rehabilitation support at home [4]. Recently developed training environments utilize not only two-dimensional video calls but also virtual reality (VR) and mixed reality (MR). These environments provide immersive training experiences that enhance motor learning through multisensory feedback (visual, auditory, and tactile) [5–7].

In Western countries, VR-based rehabilitation has also been reported to effectively improve upper limb motor function and balance after stroke. In particular, tactile and vibratory feedback targeting deep sensory input may promote motor relearning more effectively than traditional vision-based training [8]. Furthermore, the development of simple, user-friendly, and cost-effective systems is being promoted. Low-cost configurations using devices such as motion analysis systems and smartphones have already been developed [9, 10].

This study aims to integrate the research and development results of our previous telerehabilitation systems and clarify the clinical efficacy and technological feasibility of a multisensory feedback-based remote rehabilitation system. Specifically, we aim to quantitatively evaluate changes in motor performance and biometric measurements during upper limb and balance training in VR environments, as well as explore the feasibility of deploying such systems for home-based rehabilitation support.

8.1.2 Objective

This study aims to clarify the clinical efficacy and technical validity of a telerehabilitation system that utilizes multisensory feedback technology. Specifically, we aim to demonstrate how systems incorporating virtual reality (VR) and mixed reality (MR) technologies can improve motor function and ensure the continuity of rehabilitation for patients with motor paralysis due to conditions such as stroke by integratively reviewing our research findings from references [7, 11].

More specifically, we constructed a multisensory rehabilitation environment that incorporates visual display devices and auditory and vibratory stimulation devices. We then conducted system evaluations and clinical trials targeting healthy elderly individuals and persons with disabilities to verify its practical utility under remote operation. We developed a new telerehabilitation system that integrates VR technology, motion analysis devices, and vibratory stimulation devices and validated its effectiveness.

8.1.3 Methodology

In this study, we conducted an integrative analysis focusing on a prototype multisensory, feedback-based telerehabilitation application. We supplemented this analysis with findings from other related telerehabilitation projects (see Figs. 8.1 and 8.2). In reference [7], a balance evaluation and training system was developed using the built-in smartphone accelerometer, combining feedback from visual, auditory, and tactile modalities. Participants were primarily healthy elderly individuals and individuals with mild motor disabilities.

Tasks included a virtual reaching task using a motion analysis device (Kinect) and a 3D head-mounted display (3D-HMD). This setup enabled the quantitative tracking of shoulder and elbow joint movements and the evaluation of visual spatial cognitive training effectiveness. Furthermore, reference [11] examined the correlation between movement data obtained in a virtual environment (VE) and actual clinical evaluation scales. Movement quality was assessed using the Fugl-Meyer Assessment (FMA), the Wolf Motor Function Test (WMFT), the Simple Test for Evaluating Hand Function (STEF), and the Functional Balance Scale (FBS). These studies also incorporated objective evaluations using 3D motion analyses of joint movement trajectories.

Regarding communication infrastructure, real-time control was achieved using PubNub®, data transfer was facilitated via Dropbox™, and video instruction was conducted through Skype®, enabling a comprehensive assessment of the practicality of the remote system (Fig. 8.1).

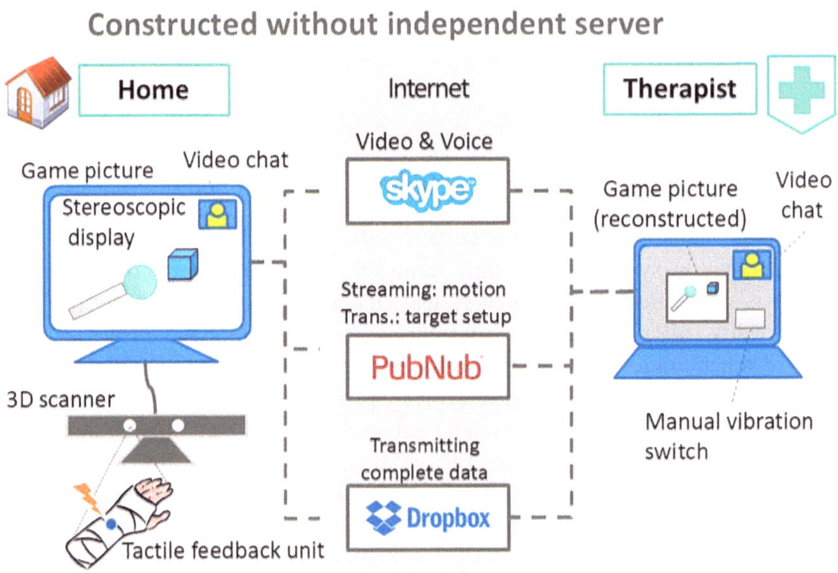

Fig. 8.1 Structure of telerehabilitation system

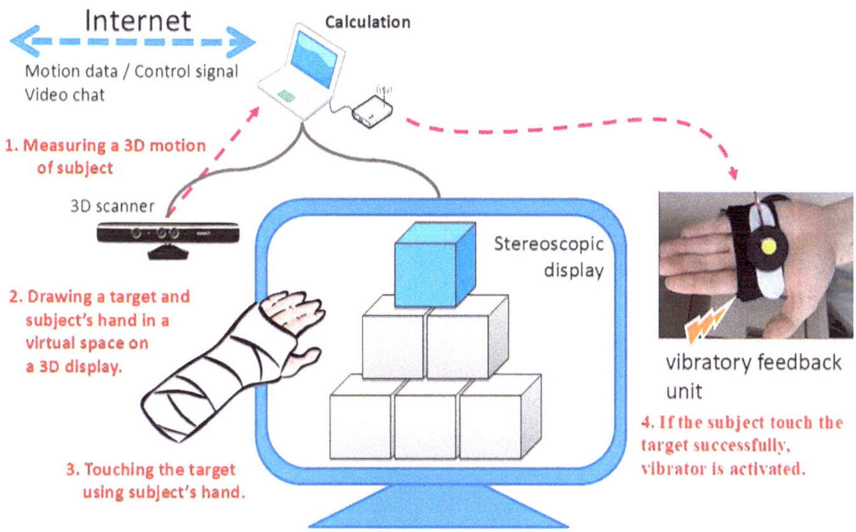

Fig. 8.2 A game "touching a target" for physical rehabilitation

8.1.4 Results

Training using VR and multisensory feedback has the potential to produce immediate and sustained effects in participants with motor paralysis. Specifically, reference [7] reported improvements in upper limb joint angles (e.g., increased shoulder flexion and reduced elbow hyperflexion) and reductions in task execution time for upper limb movement and standing balance (e.g., decreasing from 7.2 to 3.5 s and from 377 to 104 s, respectively). These outcomes are important indicators of motor learning and functional improvement.

Furthermore, real-time communication via PubNub® and data transfer through Dropbox™ were completed in under 1 minute, and video instruction via Skype® experienced no communication delays. These findings confirmed the feasibility of establishing a practical, home-based telerehabilitation environment (Fig. 8.3).

The results showed that training that incorporates integrated visual, auditory, and tactile feedback enhances participants' subjective sense of accomplishment and leads to objective improvements in motor function. Participants also expressed high satisfaction with the system's ease of operation and immediate feedback, suggesting its potential for adaptation in future home-based applications.

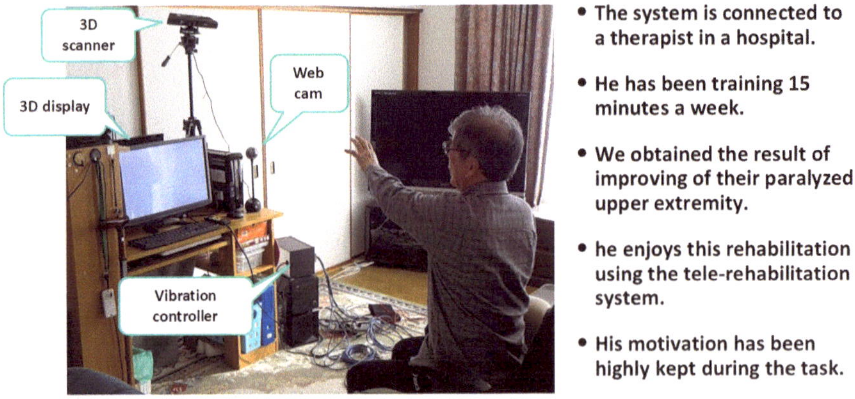

Fig. 8.3 The tele-rehabilitation system using an online connection between a hospital and a patient's home

8.1.5 Discussion

Telerehabilitation that integrates multisensory feedback has the potential to improve the efficiency of motor relearning compared to traditional, vision-centered support methods. In particular, adding vibratory stimulation enhanced deep sensory input, improving proprioception of body position and joint movement and contributing to improvements in joint angles and balance scores. These findings align with previous studies in Western countries, including those studies [9, 10] and may serve as a basis for international comparative research.

Furthermore, the affordability and widespread availability of the sensor devices and software used in this study could accelerate the social implementation of telerehabilitation. Devices such as Kinect, Skype, and Dropbox require no special environments and are easily installable in home settings. This makes them promising tools for supporting physical exercise in elderly and home care populations. Additionally, we have begun prototyping telerehabilitation systems designed for individuals with difficulty maintaining seated balance (Fig. 8.4).

However, several issues remain to be addressed, including suppressing compensatory movements, simplifying the user interface, and evaluating long-term continuity. We anticipate further development in collaboration with artificial intelligence (AI) and the Internet of Things (IoT) to create next-generation telerehabilitation systems.

Additionally, it is important to build support systems involving not only medical and welfare professionals but also family members and local communities. Progress in coordination with community-based integrated care and policy-level support could promote the institutionalization and dissemination of telerehabilitation, thereby reducing disparities in access to rehabilitation.

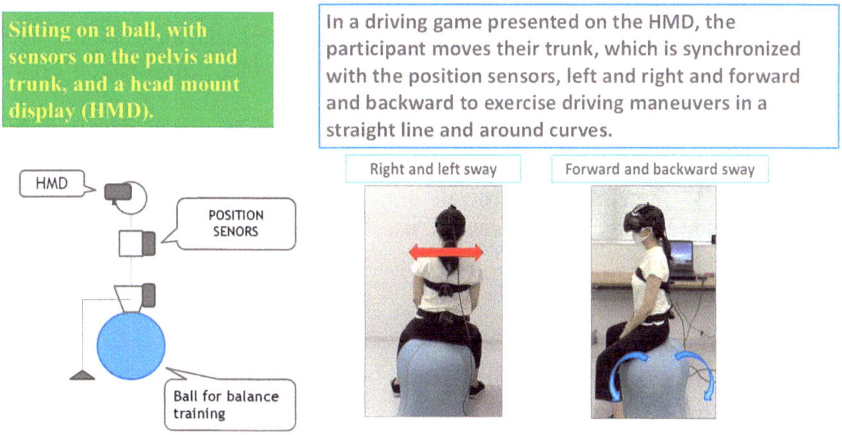

Fig. 8.4 The latest model of tele-rehabilitation for development of trunk function evaluation and training content using virtual reality

8.1.6 Conclusion

In this study, we conducted an integrated analysis of three telerehabilitation systems that utilized VR and multisensory feedback technologies. We clarified the clinical efficacy and feasibility of implementing these systems. Training environments incorporating visual, vibratory, and auditory stimuli improved motor function and balance ability among participants and demonstrated the feasibility of home-based training via ICT communication.

Notably, the use of low-cost equipment, such as Kinect and smartphones, enabled system designs suitable for home use outside of specialized facilities. This suggests a high applicability to activities of daily living (ADLs). Western studies [9, 10] also demonstrated the effectiveness of VR-based training in improving upper limb function and postural control after stroke, which supports our findings [11].

However, several challenges remain:

- Simplification of user interface (UI): User interfaces must be simplified so that they are not dependent on a mouse or keyboard and can be easily operated by elderly users.
- Control of compensatory movements: It would be beneficial to introduce posture feedback functions to prevent trunk compensation during exercises.
- Lack of long-term intervention studies: Most existing studies are short term, so the effects of continuous training on improving activities of daily living (ADLs) should be investigated.

Policy support is needed for standardization and dissemination. Training programs for professionals and insurance systems must be developed to promote widespread adoption.

Looking ahead, advanced telerehabilitation technologies integrated with AI-based automated evaluation and metaverse technologies are expected to emerge. Telerehabilitation is an important solution for expanding rehabilitation options, especially during pandemics, and it reduces disparities in access to rehabilitation. Further collaboration between clinical practice and research is essential for advancing practical rehabilitation technologies. In telerehabilitation systems, incorporating the patient's opinions is crucial for maintaining motivation. Creating telerehabilitation content that reflects the user's interests is a key factor in successful long-term engagement.

8.2 A Study of Devices for Horseback Riding Therapy for the Elderly

8.2.1 Introduction

Horseback riding therapy utilizes the walking motion of a horse to improve physical and psychological functions. While its effectiveness has been demonstrated with patients who have cerebral palsy, have had a stroke, or have autism, research focusing on elderly individuals is limited. As people age, their ability to control posture, muscle strength, and joint mobility declines. Posterior pelvic tilt and kyphotic posture are particular issues. These postural deviations may reduce safety and the therapeutic benefits of horseback riding.

Recent studies in Western countries have demonstrated that horseback riding therapy can positively impact balance, muscle strength, and mental health in older adults. For instance, Araújo et al. revealed that horseback riding therapy significantly enhanced balance and reduced the risk of falls [12]. Additionally, a meta-analysis by Zadnikar and Kastrin revealed improvements in muscle tone regulation, trunk stability, and self-efficacy [13]. However, older adults often have difficulty maintaining good posture due to kyphosis and posterior pelvic tilt, and previous studies have not sufficiently examined the use of assistive devices. The present study aimed to quantitatively and qualitatively assess the effects of a newly developed wedge-type support on the riding posture of skilled and unskilled older adults.

8.2.2 Methods

Participants included a skilled group ($n = 4$; 2 males and 2 females; mean age $= 68.8$ years; over 5 years of riding experience) and an unskilled group ($n = 4$; 2 males and 2 females; mean age $= 81.5$ years; fewer than 20 riding sessions). A trained Criollo horse (11 years old and 150 cm tall) equipped with a saddle, handles, safety stirrups, and a bridle was used for safety purposes. The

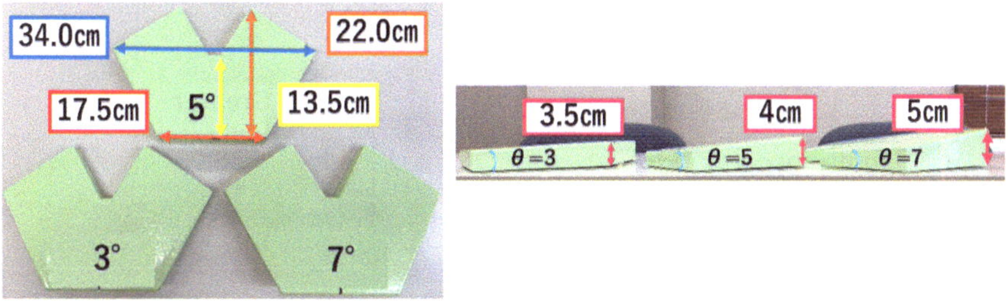

Fig. 8.5 The wedge-shaped horseback riding device in the above (left) and side (right) views

Fig. 8.6 The wedge-shaped horseback riding device installation method

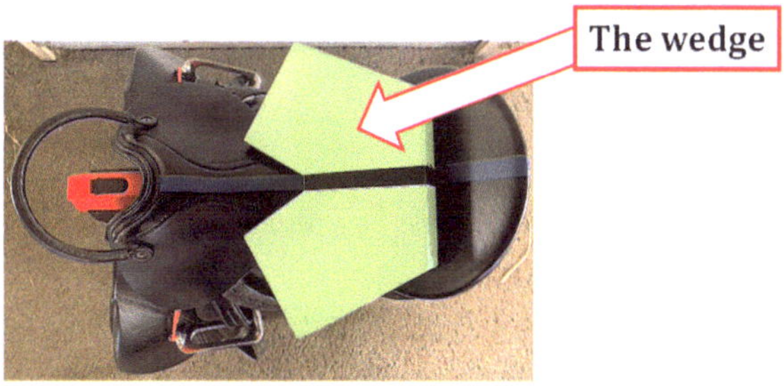

wedge-type support was made of rigid polyurethane foam and was tested under four conditions: 0°, 3°, 5°, and 7° (Figs. 8.5 and 8.6) [14].

The experiment was conducted in an indoor riding arena. The joint angles of the neck, spine, and knees were measured during straight-line and curved walking using video analysis software (Dartfish 9.0). Landmarks were identified by placing ping-pong balls on the external occipital protuberance, the spinous processes of the seventh cervical and seventh thoracic vertebrae, the greater trochanter, the lateral epicondyle of the femur, and the lateral malleolus in Figs. 8.7 and 8.8 [14].

In addition, a horseback riding therapist scored posture based on video recordings using a three-point scale (1: poor, 2: moderate, 3: good), and participants provided feedback using the System Usability Scale (SUS) [15].

8.2.3 Results

Quantitative analysis showed that skilled riders were able to maintain relatively appropriate joint angles in the neck, spine, and knees even without the device, and their posture improved further when support was used. In the unskilled group, the initial posture showed notable deviations, but with wedge support, particularly under the higher tilt conditions, the alignment of the neck, spine, and knees improved markedly.

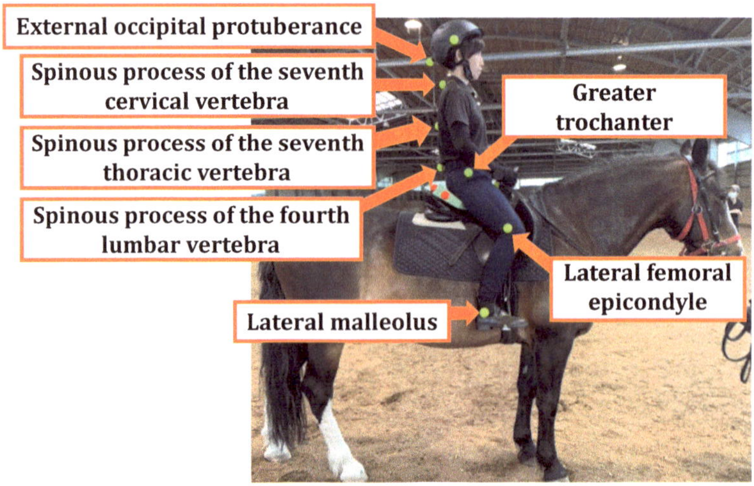

Fig. 8.7 Location of landmarks on a participant's body

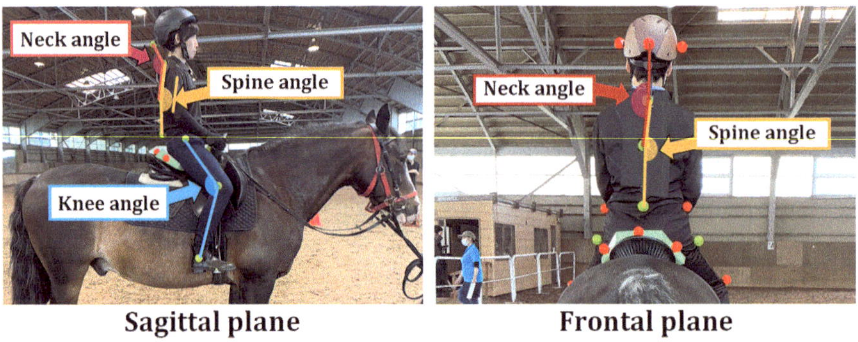

Fig. 8.8 The angles of the neck, spine, and knee joints measured by motion analysis in the sagittal and frontal planes

Qualitative assessments indicated that skilled riders consistently received good posture ratings in all conditions. Unskilled riders demonstrated clear improvements in posture, particularly with greater wedge tilt angles. The usability evaluation revealed that skilled riders reported a generally favorable score, while the unskilled group expressed high overall satisfaction. Skilled participants tended to prefer the lower wedge condition, whereas unskilled participants preferred higher wedge settings.

8.2.4 Discussion

The results confirmed that using a wedge-type support device effectively improves posture during horseback riding therapy for older adults. Skilled riders could already maintain a neutral position, but the support provided greater stability. For unskilled riders, the 5° and 7° wedges promoted anterior pelvic tilt, which facilitated neutral neck and spinal alignment and enabled a transition to better posture.

These findings align with previous Western studies. Lage et al. suggested that support devices may alter trunk and lower limb muscle activity, thereby guiding improved motor patterns [16]. Mello et al. reported that horseback riding therapy reduces blood pressure and promotes psychological relaxation in older adults [17]. Furthermore, Stergiou and Decker emphasized the importance of integrative sensory-motor approaches in enhancing dynamic balance control and noted that horseback riding therapy is a promising modality [18]. Hameed et al. demonstrated the positive effects of sensory feedback enhancement through physical interventions on posture control in older adults, which is consistent with the present findings [19].

The high SUS scores support the device's clinical applicability. Future research should comprehensively evaluate the effects of support use on muscle activity, psychological outcomes, and long-term physical function.

8.2.5 Conclusion

This study demonstrated that a prototype wedge-type postural support device effectively improved riding posture in older adults. Improvements in pelvic stability and overall postural alignment were particularly evident among unskilled participants, underscoring the device's potential utility in horseback riding therapy for the elderly population. Future studies should expand the sample size and conduct comprehensive assessments of muscle activity, balance, and psychological outcomes. Further innovations in equipment design are anticipated, including sensor-integrated saddles, wearable-linked feedback systems for posture correction, adjustable trunk-support vests, safety devices such as airbag vests and automatic-release stirrups, and the complementary use of horse simulators. Such developments are expected to advance barrier-free, inclusive design research, thereby promoting broader participation in therapeutic riding.

8.3 Reducing the Burden of Snow Removal Work: Research and Commercialization of S-Shaped Handle Shovels

8.3.1 The Necessity of Manual Snow Removal and Its Physical Toll in Snowy Regions

In snowy regions such as Hokkaido, snow removal during the winter season is essential for daily life. In some areas of Hokkaido, the average annual snowfall is between 5 and 9 m [20]. Without clearing this snow, transportation would quickly become paralyzed, and people would find it difficult to come and go or even enter and exit their homes.

However, the use of conventional snow removal tools places a significant physical burden on the body. Hardened snow is heavy, and its removal with a shovel often results in strain on the lower back and spine, leading to low back pain [21]. This burden is particularly problematic for the elderly, women, and others with limited physical strength [22].

To address this issue, a collaborative research group consisting of academia, industry, and government, including the Hokkaido Industrial Research Institute (now the Hokkaido Research Organization Industrial Research Institute), set out to develop a new snow removal tool based on ergonomic principles, aiming to reduce the physical burden on snow removal workers.

8.3.2 Development Concept

Snow removal in Hokkaido has become increasingly mechanized, with snowplows clearing roads and many households owning small snow blowers [23]. However, areas such as entrances, stairs, and gardens still require manual snow removal. The shovel, the most common manual snow removal tool, has changed little in shape since ancient times [24]. It is known to place significant stress on the lower back, and each year, many people suffer from back pain due to snow shoveling.

This study aims to reduce the physical strain of manual snow removal by improving the shovel design and enhancing the efficiency of the task. The core of the research and development process involved the analysis of snow shoveling movements using a motion analysis system to identify the causes of the physical burden, followed by efforts to reduce this burden through modifications to the shape of the shovel.

8.3.3 Measurement of Physical Load Factors Using a Motion Analysis System

A three-dimensional motion analysis system (Vicon512, Vicon Co.) was used to record the motion involved in snow shoveling. The recorded data were used to calculate the angles and joint moments of the various parts of the body. The task involved carrying and throwing a 5-kg sandbag with a shovel. In the throwing motion, the participants were instructed to aim approximately 1.5 m to the right and 1.5 m upward. Two types of handles were tested: a conventional straight handle and bent handle, as shown in Fig. 8.9.

Figure 8.10 shows the thoracic angle, and Fig. 8.11 shows the lumbar moment during the snow shoveling motion of a particular participant. The motion was divided into two phases: lifting and throwing. Immediately before lifting, the participant exhibited a complex posture involving significant flexion, lateral flexion, and rotation of the torso. After lifting the snow and adopting a slightly forward-leaning upright position, the participant swung a shovel to perform the throwing motion. Throwing involved a transition from flexion to extension, lateral flexion in the opposite direction (toward the handle), and rotation. Notably, the lateral flexion moment was greater than the flexion moment, indicating a significant left–right imbalance in the load on the lower back.

Comparisons of the thoracic angles and lumbar moments are shown in Tables 8.1 and 8.2. These tables present the thoracic angles and lumbar moments for six participants lifting 3 kg of weight using either a straight or a bent handle. Figure 8.12

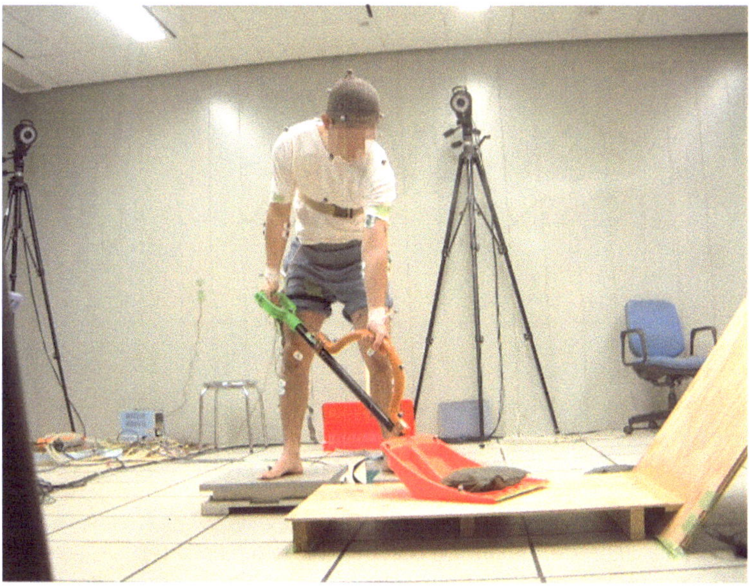

Fig. 8.9 Snow throwing experiment using a curved-handle shovel

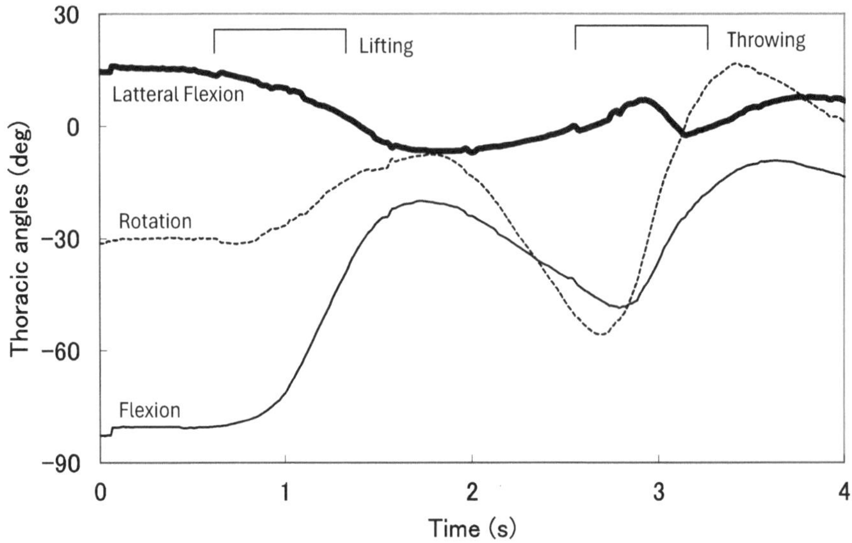

Fig. 8.10 Thorax angles during snow shoveling using a straight-handled shovel
Extension (+), right lateral flexion (+), and right axial rotation (+)

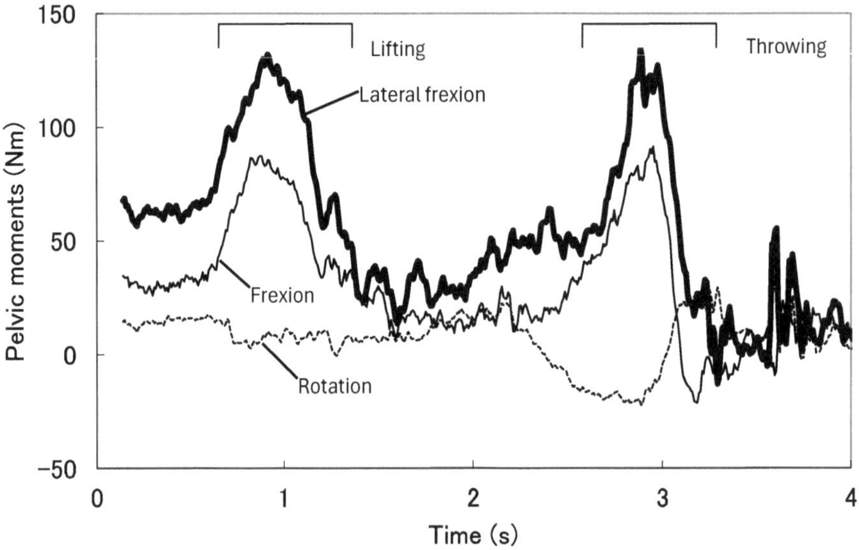

Fig. 8.11 Pelvis moments during snow shoveling using a straight-handled shovel
Extension (+), right lateral flexion (+), and right axial rotation (+)

shows the stick figures of the lifting postures for each handle type. A t-test comparison between straight and bent handles revealed that the bent handle significantly reduced flexion by 14.8° and rotation by 11.1° (Table 8.1). As shown in Table 8.2,

Table 8.1 Means and standard deviations of thoracic angle ($N = 6$)

Handle	Flexion (deg)	Lateral flexion (deg)	Rotation (deg)
Straight	83.6 ± 7.7	38.4 ± 5.2	24.2 ± 4.9
Bent	*** 68.8 ± 7.8	38.9 ± 5.3	* 13.1 ± 10.8

*$p < 0.05$; **$p < 0.01$; ***$p < 0.001$

Table 8.2 Means of standard deviations of pelvis moment ($N = 6$)

Handle	Flexion (Nm)	Lateral flexion (Nm)	Rotation (Nm)
Straight	51 ± 18	130 ± 42	57 ± 20
Bent	48 ± 11	* 111 ± 24	56 ± 16

*$p < 0.05$; **$p < 0.01$; ***$p < 0.001$

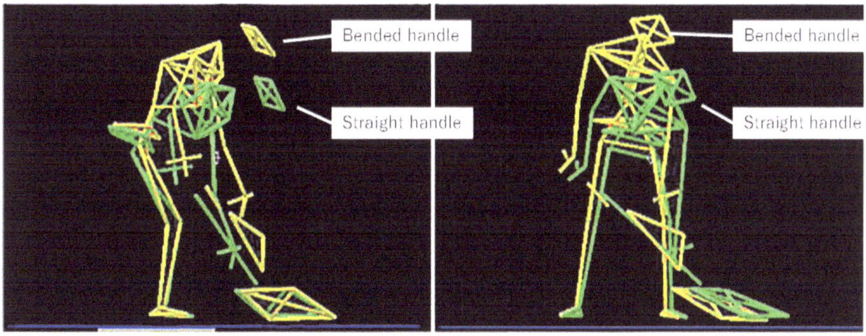

Fig. 8.12 Comparison of lifting posture using a straight-handled (green) and bent-handled (yellow) shovel
(Left: side view, right: front view)

the lateral flexion moment of the lumbar spine was reduced by 15%, indicating a reduction in the left–right imbalance of the load.

8.3.4 Analysis of Muscle Fatigue During Snow Shoveling

To analyze muscle fatigue during snow removal, a 5-min continuous snow throwing experiment was conducted. In this experiment, a slope was set up indoors, with a target positioned 1.5 m vertically and 1.5 m horizontally. Participants were instructed to throw a 3-kg sandbag toward this target every 5 s. The task was performed using two types of shovels, one with a straight handle and the other with a bent handle. Surface electromyography (EMG) sensors were placed on the left and right erector spinae muscles of each participant to measure muscle activity.

Figure 8.13 shows the normalized mean power frequency (nMPF) of the left and right erector spinae during the throwing task. The nMPF was calculated by dividing the current MPF by the initial MPF. The MPF is known to decrease with muscle

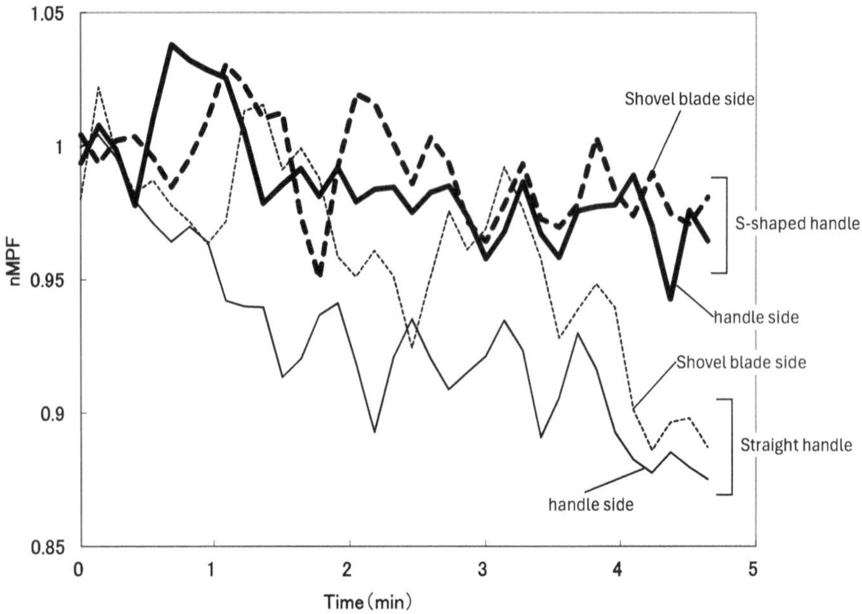

Fig. 8.13 The nMPF Plot in a 5-min throwing test

Table 8.3 Decline rate of normalized MPF

Handle	Slope [1/min]	SE	*p*
Straight	−0.0208	0.0022	<0.001
Bent	−0.0087	0.0014	

fatigue, making it a useful indicator of fatigue. The graphs illustrate that the nMPF decreased over time for both handle types, but the decline was more pronounced with the straight handle.

Table 8.3 presents the results of statistical analysis using a linear regression model to compare the rate of the nMPF decline between the two handle types. A significant difference ($p < 0.001$) was found, with the bent handle showing a lower decline rate of 0.0121 [1/min]. It is generally considered that a performance drop begins to appear when the nMPF decreases by more than 10%. For the straight handle, the nMPF dropped below 90% after 4 min, indicating substantial fatigue [25, 26]. In contrast, with the bent handle, the decline remained within 5%, suggesting that the participants could continue the task with less fatigue.

Although there was no significant difference in the nMPF decline between the left and right erector spinae over the full 5-min period, a closer look at the straight handle data revealed that up to 3.5 min, the grip side muscle (mainly activity of the erector spinae muscles on the dominant side) exhibited a greater decline. When the analysis window was limited to the first 3.5 min, a significant difference in the nMPF decline between the left and right sides was detected. This suggests that with the straight handle, there was asymmetry in fatigue, with the grip side (the side used to pull up the snow) experiencing more intense fatigue. After 3.5 min, it was assumed that participants adjusted their movement strategy to rely more on the bucket side muscle (mainly activity of the erector spinae muscles on the nondominant side), which had experienced less fatigue.

8.3.5 Evaluation of Handle Shape

To this point, it has been demonstrated that the bent handle shovel contributes to improved posture, reduced fatigue in the erector spinae muscles, and decreased lumbar moments. However, for commercialization, it is necessary to evaluate the design usability. Therefore, four prototype shovel handles with posture-improving features comparable to those of the bent handle, specifically designed to reduce trunk flexion, were fabricated, as shown in Fig. 8.14. A subjective usability evaluation was conducted.

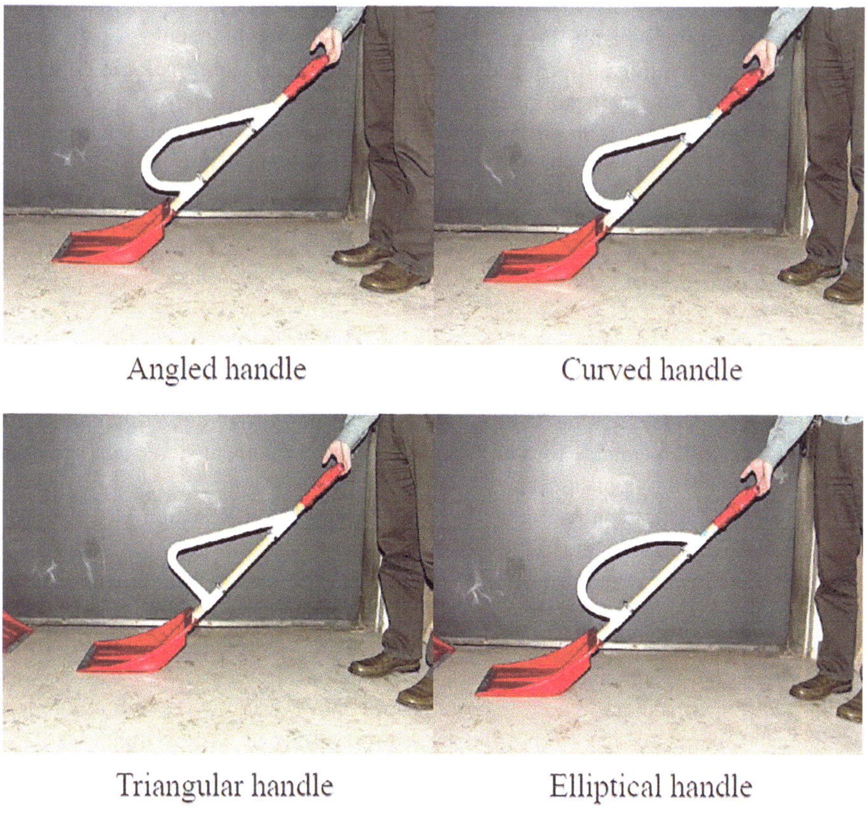

Fig. 8.14 Shovel handles used in usability experiment

Table 8.4 Subjective ratings of shovel handle usability compared to the straight handle

Handle	Grip comfort	Ease of lifting	Ease of throwing	Average
Straight	3.0 ± 0.0	3.0 ± 0.0	3.0 ± 0.0	3.0
Angled	*** 3.9 ± 0.6	*** 4.2 ± 0.6	*** 4.0 ± 0.6	4.1
Curved	** 3.9 ± 0.5	*** 4.0 ± 0.6	** 4.3 ± 0.7	4.1
Triangular	** 3.8 ± 0.6	*** 3.9 ± 0.9	*** 3.9 ± 0.5	3.9
Elliptical	*** 3.9 ± 1.1	*** 4.1 ± 0.9	*** 3.6 ± 0.8	3.9

Participants rated the usability of each shovel handle on a five-point Likert scale, with 3 as the baseline score for the straight handle (neutral), 1 = very poor, and 5 = very good. Dunnett's multiple comparison test was performed to assess differences from the straight handle
*$p < 0.05$; **$p < 0.01$; ***$p < 0.001$

The evaluation included the following three criteria: grip comfort, ease of lifting, and ease of throwing. Ratings were given on a five-point Likert scale (1 = very poor, 5 = very good), with the straight-handled shovel set as the baseline, with a score of 3. Dunnett's multiple comparison test was applied to assess statistical differences in usability scores. Seven participants were included in this evaluation.

The results of the usability evaluation are shown in Table 8.4. All four handle types received significantly higher scores than the straight handle for all three categories: grip comfort, lifting, and throwing. A separate Holm multiple comparison test revealed no significant differences among the four handle types. Therefore, among the angled and curved handles that had the highest average scores, the simpler curved handle was selected as the model for commercialization.

8.3.6 Conclusion

Based on the results of this study, a snow shovel designed to reduce physical strain was successfully commercialized (Fig. 8.15). The handle on the bucket side was bent into a large S-shape, creating a form equivalent to that of the curved handle. This shovel is currently available for purchase at home improvement stores across Japan and is widely used by consumers.

The S-shaped snow shovel developed by the Hokkaido Research Organization Industrial Research Institute achieved a significant breakthrough in reducing the burden on the lower back during snow removal. Its commercialization and recognition through the Good Design Award—one of Japan's most prestigious design evaluation and commendation programs—demonstrate the social acknowledgment of its innovative design and user-centered approach [27].

In addition to standard snow removal, other shovel variations, such as models with bucket shapes specialized for disaster recovery, have also been commercialized and are receiving positive feedback in the market. Continued research and development in this field are expected to contribute to safer and more comfortable snow removal practices in the future.

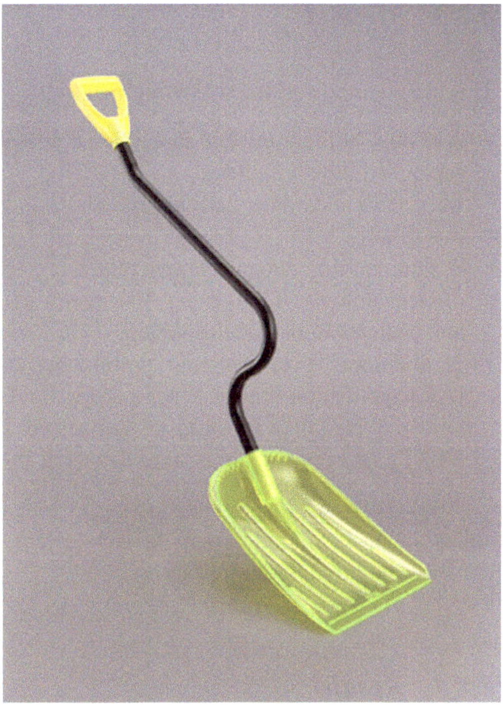

Fig. 8.15 Bent shaft grip polycarbonate snow shovel

8.4 Barrier-Free Housing for Fall Prevention in the Elderly

8.4.1 Background and Objectives

In Japan, people aged 65 and over account for 29.3% of the total population [28], and falls and fractures rank among the top three causes of individuals requiring nursing care, highlighting the seriousness of the issue [29]. Notably, approximately 60% of fall-related deaths—excluding those in unspecified locations—occur in the home [30], indicating the significant impact of the residential environment. However, many existing homes remain inadequately barrier-free. Although government subsidies are available for home renovations, actual implementation has not kept pace.

This paper aims to present:

1. An overview of policy comparisons between Japan and other countries (the UK, the USA, and Nordic countries).
2. The identification of fall risk factors in Japanese homes based on a six-type classification of falls.
3. An analysis of renovation case studies conducted by the Institute of Gerontology (IOG).
4. An examination of methods for visualizing fall risks using an augmented reality (AR) application.

8.4.2 Methods

This study employed the following methods:

- A review of literature and institutional policies on housing and fall prevention in Japan and other countries.
- Interviews and home visit surveys conducted with patients who were hospitalized due to falls.
- A comparative analysis of three renovation case studies conducted by the Institute of Gerontology (IOG), using floor plans, assessments of daily living conditions, and changes in physical function.
- A functional overview and preliminary evaluation of an augmented reality (AR) application jointly developed by the University of Tokyo, Osaka University, the National Institute of Advanced Industrial Science and Technology (AIST), and the Nikken Sekkei Research Institute.

All surveys and development activities were conducted through multidisciplinary collaboration involving experts in architecture, information engineering, medicine, nursing, and rehabilitation sciences.

8.4.3 Results

8.4.3.1 Comparison of Housing Renovation Policies for General Residences in Japan and Western Countries

In Japan, small-scale home renovations for elderly individuals are subsidized through the Ministry of Health, Labour and Welfare's Long-Term Care Insurance system [31]. However, these subsidies are limited to post-incident renovations after the need for care arises, and preventive renovations have not become widespread.

In the UK, the "Lifetime Neighbourhoods" initiative incorporates barrier-free housing renovation into the broader framework of creating age-friendly communities [32]. Comprehensive design strategies include not only barrier removal and handrail installation but also improvements to outdoor spaces and sidewalks. The Disabled Facilities Grant (DFG) provides up to £30,000 for home renovations—including both owner-occupied and rental properties—depending on local authority policies and household income levels [33].

In the USA, renovation assistance varies by state. While there are no nationwide programs, Medicaid home- and community-based services (HCBS) offer support that enables eligible individuals to remain in their homes and communities instead of entering institutional care settings [34].

In Nordic countries, universal design is mandated even in private residential construction from the planning stage. Features such as stairways, entrances, and bathrooms are designed accordingly from the outset [35, 36].

The situation in each country is summarized in Table 8.5.

Table 8.5 International comparison of home modification support systems for the elderly

Country/ region	Program/policy name	Target population	Scope of support	Maximum grant/funding	Administering body	Key features
Japan	Long-Term Care Insurance (介護保険による住宅改修補助)	Certified care recipients (support or care level)	Handrails, step elimination, nonslip flooring, etc.	¥200,000 (90% public subsidy)	Local governments (under MHLW)	Individual-based, medical-care linked, needs assessment by care managers
UK	Disabled Facilities Grant (DFG)	The elderly and people with disabilities	Bathroom/kitchen modifications, ramps, widening doors, etc.	£30,000 (England)	Local authorities	Mandatory legal scheme; based on OT assessment; integrated with health and housing policy
USA	Medicaid HCBS Waivers	Low-income seniors	Structural modifications, ramps, stairlifts, accessible bathrooms	Varies by state	State Medicaid agencies	State-specific programs; significant support for veterans; needs based
Sweden (Nordics)	Bostadsanpassningsbidrag (Housing Adaptation Grant)	Seniors or individuals with functional limitations	Door widening, bathroom redesign, height-adjustable fixtures	No fixed cap; based on individual need	Municipalities	Individualized support; based on OT and medical certification; part of universal welfare

8.4.3.2 Exploring Causes of Falls in Japanese Homes and Preventive Measures Using Renovations and Technology

From 2017 to 2020, the authors conducted interviews and home visit surveys targeting community-dwelling older adults who had been hospitalized due to falls and sustained proximal femoral fractures. These investigations aimed to understand the circumstances surrounding the falls, assess the condition of the home environment, and evaluate the status of housing renovations. Based on the findings from the fall situation assessments, falls were classified into six categories, primarily to inform architectural fall prevention strategies. Subsequent home visits examined whether the renovations contributed to fall prevention and whether the home environment supported continued residence over the long term. In addition, the study explored the visualization of fall risks using advanced technology and initiated the development of an application designed to assist medical and welfare professionals in implementing fall prevention measures.

Six Categories of Falls and Corresponding Architectural Measures

Based on research by Imaeda et al., falls within the home can be classified into six categories (Fig. 8.16) [37]:

A. Stumbling.
B. Missing a step.
C. Slipping.

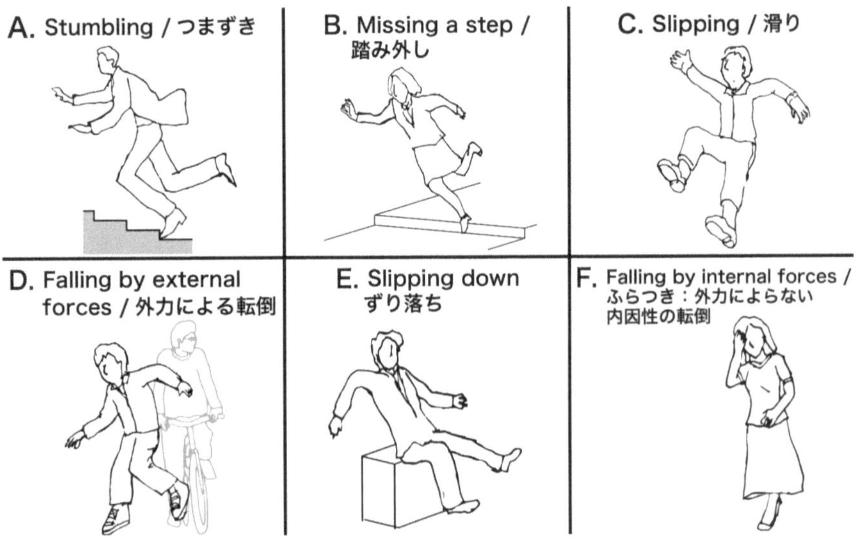
A. Stumbling / つまずき
B. Missing a step / 踏み外し
C. Slipping / 滑り
D. Falling by external forces / 外力による転倒
E. Slipping down ずり落ち
F. Falling by internal forces / ふらつき：外力によらない 内因性の転倒

Fig. 8.16 Definition of falls: fall model

D. Falling by external forces.
E. Slipping down.
F. Fall by internal forces.

Corresponding architectural interventions include level elimination, installation of handrails, use of nonslip flooring, high-visibility lighting, improved furniture layout, and appropriate height settings. These strategies were applied in actual renovation case studies during the home visit surveys, showing that risk classification led to effective design proposals.

Home Visit Surveys

From 2017 to 2020, the authors conducted a study in collaboration with the Institute of Gerontology (IOG) at the University of Tokyo and the University of Tokyo Hospital, targeting 43 patients who had been hospitalized due to proximal femoral fractures. Home visits were also conducted with 23 of these patients after discharge. The study focused on changes in patients' physical function (assessed using the GLFS-25), the circumstances of their falls, changes in their home environment, and the level of support provided by family members. As a result, a variety of housing renovation cases were identified, as described below [38]:

- No. 1: Handrails originally installed for the husband were supplemented with additional rails for the patient in the bathroom and living room. Since the patient had multiple conditions and already used the living room as a bedroom, the renovation was relatively smooth (Fig. 8.17).
- No. 2: Despite the onset of dementia after discharge, extensive renovations were realized with support from the daughter, who visited regularly from afar. Modifications included flooring changes, conversion of the toilet from Japanese to Western style, complete renovation of the bathroom, kitchen, and washroom, removal of level differences, and handrails at the entrance. However, some new installations caused confusion due to the patient's cognitive decline (Fig. 8.18).
- No. 3: The patient already had dementia, and the daughter's family expanded the toilet and added handrails in the toilet and entrance, improving caregiving accessibility (Fig. 8.19).
- No. 4: The building had been rebuilt in 2007, and only bedding was changed from a futon to a bed. Handrails had already been installed in response to previous family members' health conditions (Fig. 8.20).
- No. 5: The patient had already renovated the home for her late husband 10 years earlier. No additional modifications were needed after her own fall, demonstrating the long-term benefit of prior renovations (Fig. 8.21).

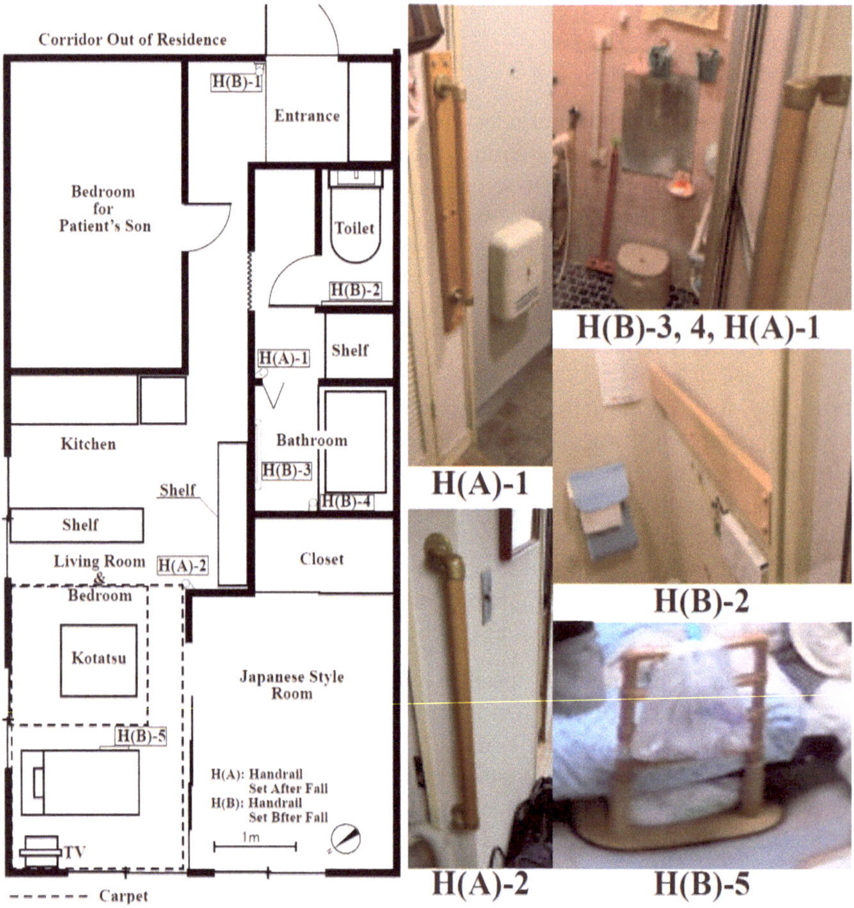

Fig. 8.17 No. 1 Floor plan and handrails

These cases illustrate that the necessity and scale of renovation are greatly influenced by the patient's cognitive status, existing facilities, and the availability of family support. Particularly for individuals with dementia, new installations or environmental changes may cause confusion, highlighting the importance of balancing "safety" and "familiarity" in design.

Additionally, family involvement—such as proposing renovations, sharing costs, and monitoring—plays a vital role in post-discharge living continuity. This reconfirms the need to integrate architectural (hardware) and welfare (software) support.

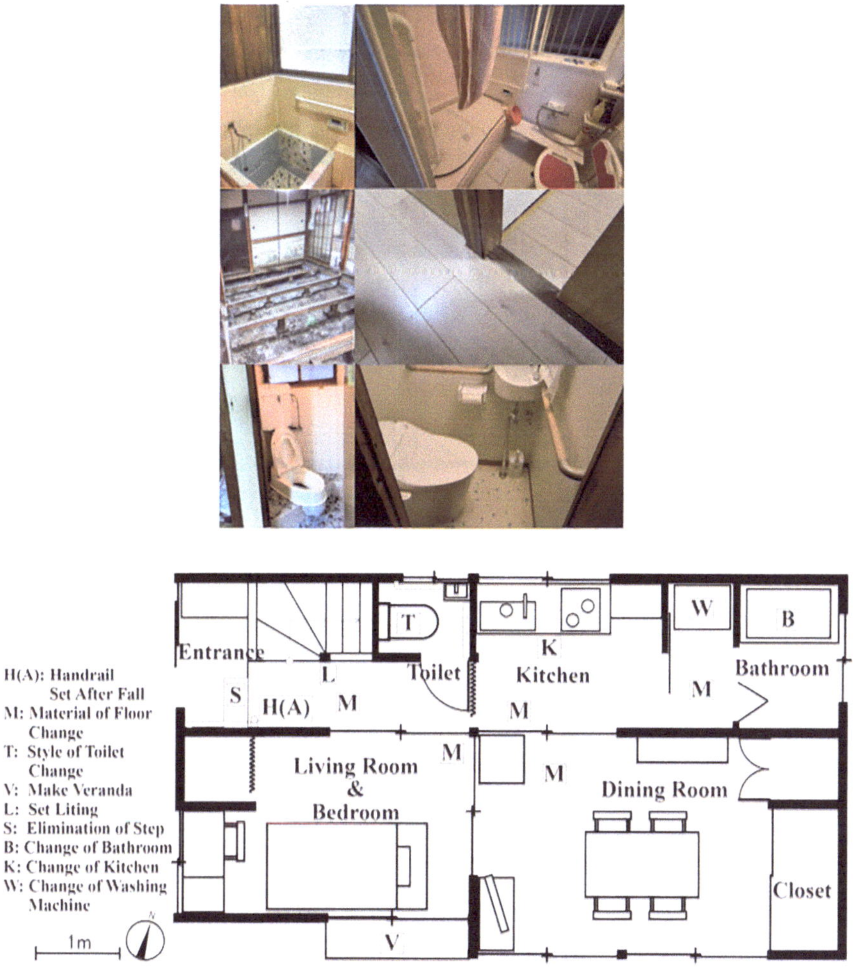

Fig. 8.18 Before and after repair in No. 2 (bathroom, living room, toilet) and floor plan

Technological Evaluation of Fall Risk: AR-Based Risk Visualization

Many home renovations are carried out by medical and welfare professionals without architectural expertise. Our surveys confirmed that architectural professionals rarely intervened, and differences in knowledge and experience among welfare workers often led to inconsistent measures. In response, a collaborative team developed a smartphone-based AR application that scans the home and displays fall risks in real time. Future enhancements will include fall risk customization based on physical status (using the same camera) and features for suggesting renovation solutions such as handrail placement, level elimination, and furniture layout changes [39] (Fig. 8.22).

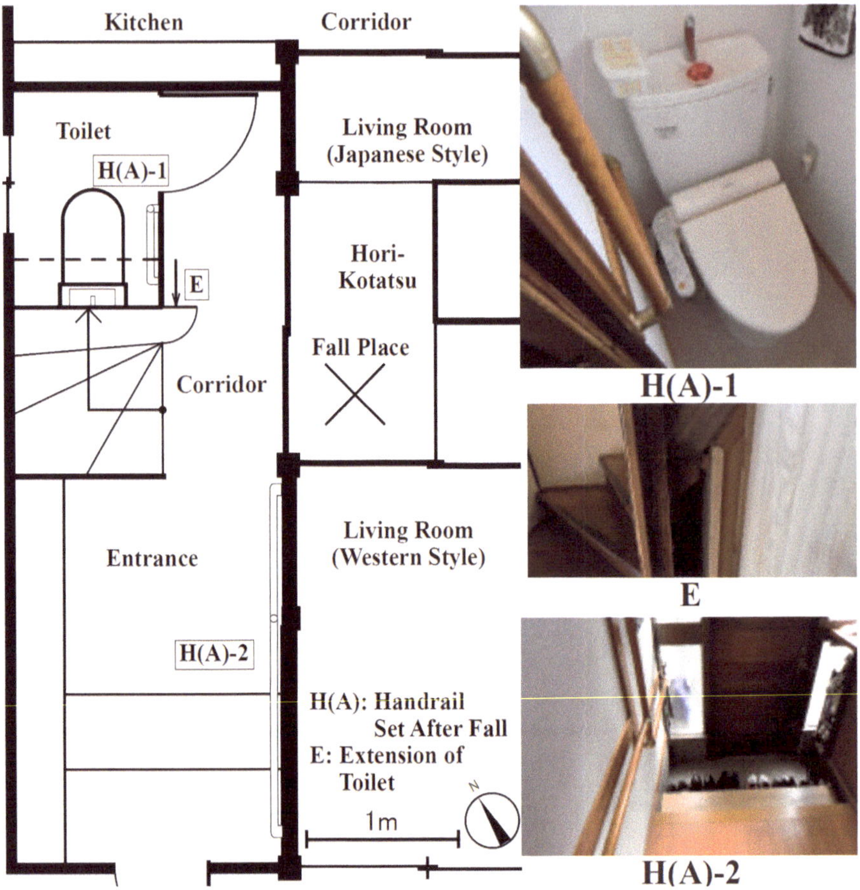

Fig. 8.19 No. 3 Floor plan and repair

8.4.4 Discussion

Architectural intervention requires design considerations based on residents' behavioral patterns as well as their cognitive and physical functions. Simply removing physical barriers is not sufficient; rather, it is essential to understand how individuals navigate and interact with their environment—such as habitual pathways, visual perception, and daily routines. In addition to handrails and the elimination of level differences, spatial layout, lighting design, surface textures, and furniture arrangement all play a critical role in creating a safe and navigable environment, particularly for individuals with impaired vision or reduced mobility.

The AR application currently under development provides an innovative support tool for professionals in the medical, welfare, and architectural fields. By enabling real-time identification of potential fall risks through smartphone-based scanning, it

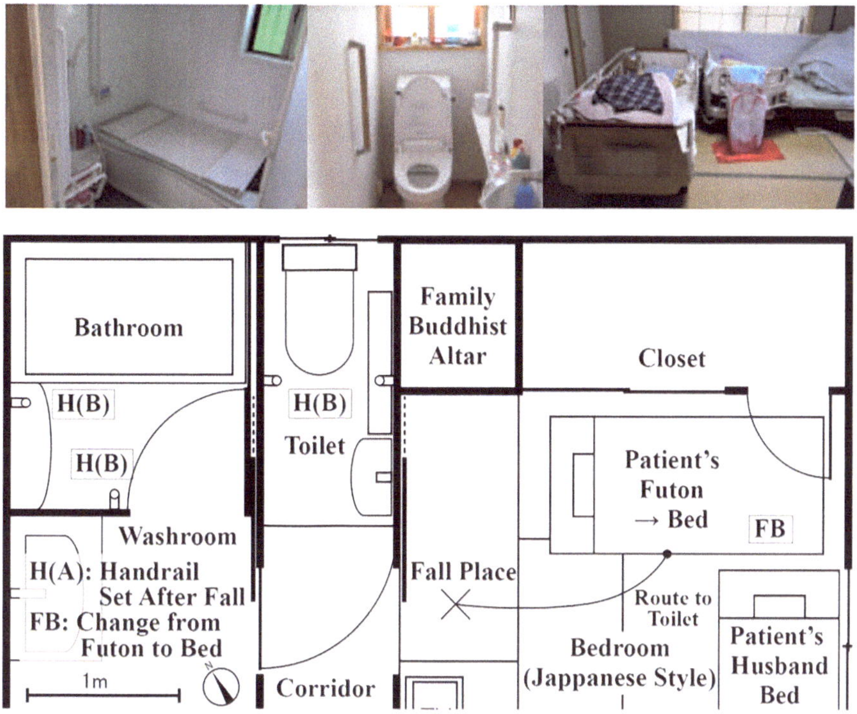

Fig. 8.20 No. 4 Plan and repair

facilitates multidisciplinary planning of personalized renovation strategies tailored to residents' physical and cognitive abilities. However, to ensure the app's effectiveness and broader adoption, special attention must be given to its usability—particularly for the older adults and nontechnical staff—as well as to privacy concerns, especially when scanning and storing data from private living spaces.

8.4.5 Conclusion

Properly executed housing renovations play a critical role in fall prevention and support elderly individuals in continuing to live safely and independently in their familiar home environments. These renovations not only reduce immediate physical risks but also contribute to maintaining dignity, autonomy, and quality of life. Especially for those with cognitive decline or limited family support, well-designed homes can serve as a stable foundation for aging in place.

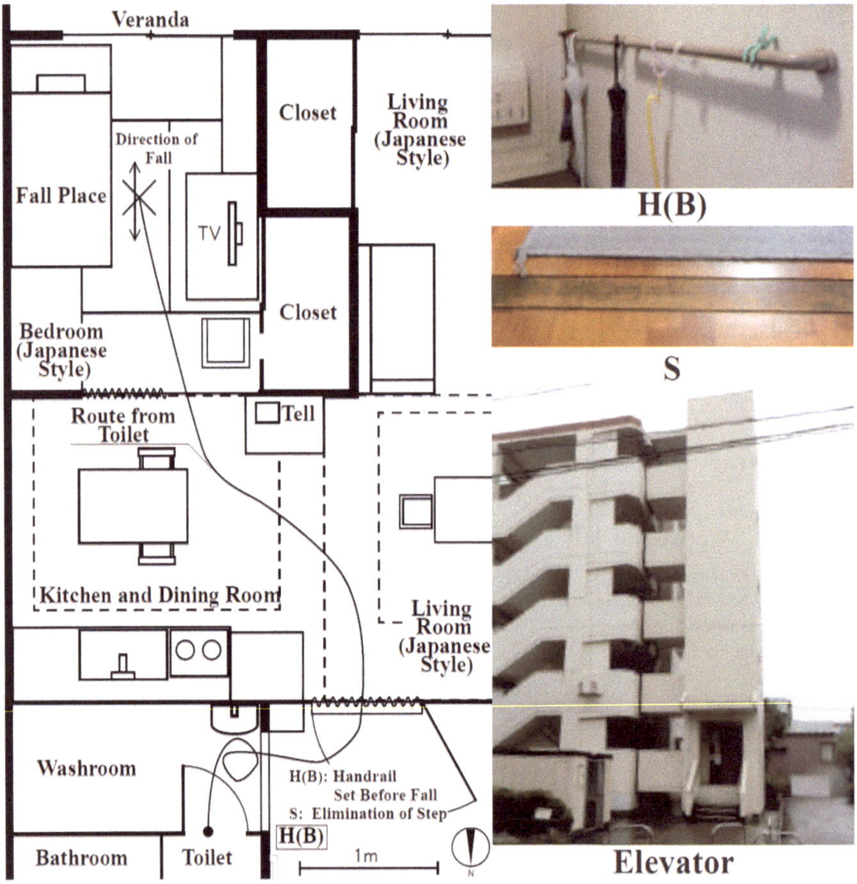

Fig. 8.21 No. 5 Floor plan and repair

Future policy frameworks should shift from reactive, post-incident interventions to proactive, preventive renovation schemes. To achieve this, it is essential to establish standardized guidelines for fall risk assessments, promote interdisciplinary collaboration, and ensure that financial and technical support mechanisms are in place for individuals and families across diverse socioeconomic backgrounds.

The case studies from the Institute of Gerontology (IOG) and the development of the AR application provide a promising, evidence-based model for integrating architecture, welfare, and technology. These initiatives demonstrate the potential for personalized and scalable fall prevention strategies and should be expanded, refined, and institutionalized nationwide to meet the growing needs of an aging population.

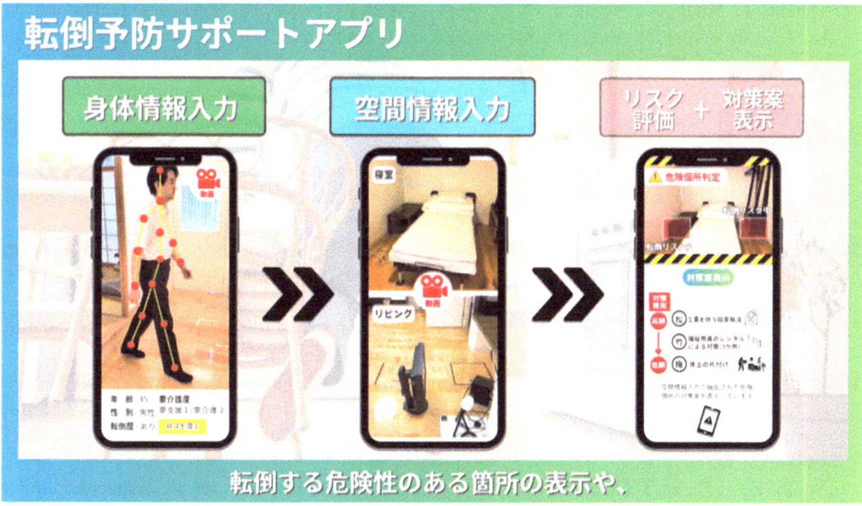

Fig. 8.22 AR application under development

References

1. Ministry of Health, Labour and Welfare: White Paper on the Aging Society (2023). Retrieved from https://www8.cao.go.jp/kourei/whitepaper/index-w.html
2. Tsutsui, T.: The current state and future development of the long-term care insurance system in Japan. J. Natl. Inst. Public Health. **59**, 372–379 (2010)
3. Hatano, E.: Long-term care insurance in Japan: How physicians are involved in providing rehabilitation for the elderly. JMAJ. **55**(3), 231–239 (2012)
4. Kairy, D., Lehoux, P., Vincent, C., Visintin, M.: A systematic review of clinical outcomes, clinical process, healthcare utilization, and costs associated with telerehabilitation. Disabil. Rehabil. **31**(6), 427–447 (2009)
5. Weiss, P. L. (T.), Keshner, E. A., & Levin, M. F. (Eds.). Virtual reality for physical and motor rehabilitation. Springer Science + Business Media. (2014) https://doi.org/10.1007/978-1-4939-0968-1
6. Tanaka, T., Shirogane, S., Maeda, Y., et al.: Effectiveness of a new combined system using a force plate and vibratory stimulation device for balance training in patients with stroke. In: Proceedings of the 1st International Conference on Applied Bionics and Biomechanics (2010). https://doi.org/10.1109/SI.2009.5384551
7. Kato, N., Tanaka, T., Sugihara, S., Shimizu, K.: Development and evaluation of a new telerehabilitation system based on VR technology using multisensory feedback for patients with stroke. J. Phys. Ther. Sci. **27**(10), 3185–3190 (2015)
8. Eckhouse, R.H., Morash, R.P., Maulucci, R.A.: Sensory feedback and the impaired motor system. J. Med. Syst. **14**(2), 93–105 (1990)
9. Holden, M.K., Dyar, T.A., Dayan-Cimadoro, L.: Telerehabilitation using a virtual environment improves upper extremity function in patients with stroke. IEEE Trans. Neural Syst. Rehabil. Eng. **15**(1), 36–42 (2007)
10. Ustinova, K.I., Leonard, W.A., Cassavaugh, N.D., Ingersoll, C.D.: Development of a 3D immersive video game to improve arm-postural coordination in patients with TBI. J. Neuroeng. Rehabil. **8**, 61 (2011)

11. Tanaka, T., Kudo, A., Sugihara, S., Izumi, T., Maeda, Y., Kato, N., Miyasaka, T., Holden, M. K.: A study on the relationship between upper limb training and clinical evaluation in a virtual environment. J. Phys. Ther. Sci. **25**(5), 575–580 (2013). https://doi.org/10.1589/jpts.25.575
12. Araujo, T.B., Silva, R.A., Costa, J.N., et al.: Effects of horseback riding therapy on balance and mobility in older adults: A randomized controlled trial. Geriatr Gerontol Int. **21**(5), 412–418 (2021)
13. Zadnikar, M., Kastrin, A.: Effects of hippotherapy and therapeutic horseback riding on postural control or balance in children with cerebral palsy: A meta-analysis. Dev. Med. Child Neurol. **53**(8), 684–691 (2011)
14. Miura, R., Esashi, N., Mitani, A., Miura, T., Tanaka, T.: Posture retention devices for older adults undergoing horseback riding therapy. COJ Nurse Healthc. **9**(1), 939–946 (2024). https://doi.org/10.31031/COJNH.2024.09.0007044
15. Brooke, J.: SUS: A "quick and dirty" usability scale. In: Jordan, et al. (eds.) Usability Evaluation in Industry, pp. 189–194. Taylor & Francis, London (1996)
16. Lage, J.B., Ribeiro, M.F., Teixeira, V.d.P.A., Rosa, R.C., Ferreira, A.A., Espindula, A.P.: Effect of horse riding equipment in activity of trunk and lower limb muscles in equine-assisted therapy. Acta Sci. Health Sci. **42**(1), e52739 (2020). https://doi.org/10.4025/actascihealthsci.v42i1.52739
17. Mello, E.C., Diniz, L.H., Lage, J.B., Monteiro, V.S., Ribeiro, M.F., et al.: Impact of equine assisted therapy on the cardiovascular parameters of the elderly. ABCS Health Sci. **46**, e021216 (2021). https://doi.org/10.7322/abcshs.2019161.1430
18. Stergiou, N., Decker, L.M.: Human movement variability, nonlinear dynamics, and pathology: Is there a connection? Hum. Mov. Sci. **30**(5), 869–888 (2011)
19. Hameed, S., Iqbal, Z., Khan, M., et al.: Sensory feedback interventions for improving balance in older adults: A systematic review. Clin. Interv. Aging. **17**, 221–235 (2022)
20. Japan Meteorological Agency.: Historical weather data. Available from: https://www.data.jma.go.jp/stats/etrn/
21. Nadler, S.F., Malanga, G.A., Bartoli, L.A., Feinberg, J.H., Prybicien, M., Deprince, M.: Hip muscle imbalance and low back pain in athletes: Influence of core strengthening. Med. Sci. Sports Exerc. **34**(1), 9–16 (2002)
22. Kinoshita, H., Obuchi, S., Umezu, Y.: Snow shoveling-related low back pain in the elderly: Epidemiological and biomechanical perspectives. Geriatr Gerontol Int. **11**(3), 361–369 (2011)
23. Aoki, K., Takahashi, H.: Snow and ice control in Japan: Policy and technical approaches. In: Proceedings of the 20th International Road Federation World Meeting (2012)
24. Nagano, H., Begg, R.: Biomechanical analysis of snow shoveling to evaluate musculoskeletal loading and ergonomic interventions. Appl. Ergon. **44**(1), 151–158 (2013)
25. De Luca, C.J.: Myoelectric manifestations of localized muscular fatigue in humans. Crit. Rev. Biomed. Eng. **11**(4), 251–279 (1984)
26. Dimitrov, G.V., Arabadzhiev, T.I., Mileva, K.N., Bowtell, J.L., Crichton, N., Dimitrova, N.A.: Muscle fatigue during dynamic contractions assessed by new spectral indices. Med. Sci. Sports Exerc. **38**(11), 1971–1979 (2006)
27. Good Design Award: 2008. Available from: https://www.g-mark.org/
28. Cabinet Office Japan: Annual Report on the Aging Society in 2025, 2025 (in Japanese)
29. Ministry of Health, Labour and Welfare (MHLW).: Overview of the 2022 National Livelihood Survey
30. e-Stat, Statistics of Japan: Vital statistics (confirmed figures and archived tables): number of deaths due to accidental causes other than traffic accidents (codes W00–X59) by age group, cause (three-digit ICD-10 code), sex, and place of occurrence
31. Ministry of Health, Labour and Welfare: Home renovations under long-term care insurance. https://www.mhlw.go.jp/general/seido/toukatsu/suishin/dl/07.pdf
32. UK Department for Communities and Local Government: Lifetime neighbourhoods. https://assets.publishing.service.gov.uk/media/5a79d58e40f0b66d161ae79b/2044122.pdf (2011)

33. UK Government: Disabled Facilities Grant (DFG). https://www.gov.uk/disabled-facilities-grants (2023)
34. Medicaid.gov: Home and community-based services (HCBS). https://www.medicaid.gov/medicaid/home-community-based-services
35. Lidelöw, H., et al.: A review of accessibility regulations in building codes: Nordic examples. Scand. J. Public Health. (2013) https://journals.sagepub.com/doi/10.1177/1403494813500860
36. Norwegian Building Code Regulation (TEK17). Chapter 12–3: Universal Design in New Housing. https://lovdata.no/dokument/SF/forskrift/2017-06-19-840/KAPITTEL_12-3#%C2%A712-18
37. Imaeda, S., et al.: Characteristics of fall places and injuries in Omuta city by analyzed ambulance dispatch data 2016. J. Archit. Plann., AIJ. **84**(759), 1077–1087 (2019). https://doi.org/10.3130/aija.84.1077
38. Imaeda, S., Son, B.-K., Uchiyama, E., Tanaka, T., Taniguchi, S., Unyaporn, S., Miyoshi, Y., Tanaka, T., Iijima, K., Otsuki, T.: The architectural factors in continuity of living for the elderly after falls and fractures. In: The 12th International Symposium on Architectural Interchanges in Asia, Pyeongchang, Korea, pp. 420–424 (2018)
39. Imaeda, S., et al.: Designing an application prototype for fall risk evaluation in housing with multi-disciplinary researchers. In: The 10th Annual Scientific Meeting of the Japanese Society for Fall Prevention (2023)

Chapter 9
Supporting Communication for Individuals with Speech and Hearing Disorders

Ken-ichiro Yabu, Takahiro Miura, and Toshiaki Tanaka

Abstract This chapter discusses support measures for language disorders in the first section and for hearing impairments in the second section. Section 9.1: Human speech is not only used for verbal communication but also for a wide variety of purposes, such as singing and music expression, mimicking, sensing information from tone, and inducing laughter. They play important roles in the expression and dignity of a person and contribute significantly to facilitating human relationships. Therefore, patients who have lost their voice due to laryngectomy for laryngeal cancer or other cancers have a significant psychological impact and may tend to withdraw. In this chapter, an overview of the classification of speech disorders is first described, and then supporting technologies and approaches currently in practical use are introduced. Subsequently, the research attempted by the authors is introduced. It would be great if a viewpoint that shows a direction for future research on assistive technology for speech disorders could be shared with readers.

Section 9.2: Information accessibility for deaf and hard of hearing (DHH) individuals has evolved significantly from traditional hearing aids to comprehensive digital solutions. This chapter examines contemporary approaches to information acquisition support for the DHH community, encompassing 1.5 billion people worldwide with varying degrees of hearing loss. We review three primary categories of assistive technologies: hearing enhancement devices, including hearing aids and

K. Yabu
Research Center for Advanced Science and Technology, The University of Tokyo, Tokyo, Japan

Institute of Gerontology, The University of Tokyo, Tokyo, Japan
e-mail: yabu@g.ecc.u-tokyo.ac.jp

T. Miura
Research Institute on Human and Societal Augmentation (RIHSA), National Institute of Advanced Industrial Science and Technology (AIST), Chiba, Japan
e-mail: miura-t@aist.go.jp

T. Tanaka (✉)
Research Center for Advanced Science and Technology/Institute of Gerontology, The University of Tokyo, Tokyo, Japan
e-mail: t.tanaka@iog.u-tokyo.ac.jp; tanaka@bfp.rcast.u-tokyo.ac.jp

T. Tanaka (ed.), *Inclusive and Barrier-Free Designs for Rehabilitation Engineering*,
https://doi.org/10.1007/978-981-95-5783-7_9

cochlear implants with wireless transmission capabilities; real-time captioning systems utilizing speech recognition and respeak methods for live broadcasts and educational settings; and communication support applications that facilitate intercommunication between speech, text, and sign language. The chapter also explores specialized applications in educational environments and sports participation, highlighting evidence-based practices and emerging technologies. While technological advances have remarkably improved accessibility through smartphone applications and remote captioning systems, substantial challenges remain in ensuring universal access and maintaining high accuracy across diverse communication preferences. Future developments must address the heterogeneous needs of DHH communities while respecting both individual communication choices and deaf cultural values in designing inclusive information systems.

9.1 Supporting for Speech Disorders

9.1.1 Technology to Support Speech and Language Disorders

9.1.1.1 The Variability of Speech Disorders

As suggested by the wide variety of voice functions, there are many different types of speech disorders. This is because various physical organs associated with speech can cause disorders. The degree of impairment ranges from mild to severe. The required needs also vary from person to person, depending on the type and degree of disability. Therefore, various methods exist to support speech communication. It is necessary to note such variety when studying assistive technologies and to be aware of what kind of needs it is intended to be applied to.

First, the mechanism of human speech is described. Human speech is (1) a breath exhaled from the lungs into the trachea, (2) the vocal cords vibrate to produce the primary laryngeal sound, and (3) the primary laryngeal sound is characterized by resonance in the vocal tract and is produced as speech containing linguistic information. If any of these processes are impaired, it is difficult to speak normally, and different support methods are required for each cause.

As an example of classification, the following three categories of speech and language disorder were used according to the criteria for recognition of physical disability by Japan's Ministry of Health, Labour and Welfare.

(a) Disorders of articulation or voice
(b) Aphasia
(c) Disorder due to hearing impairment

This is schematically illustrated in Fig. 9.1.

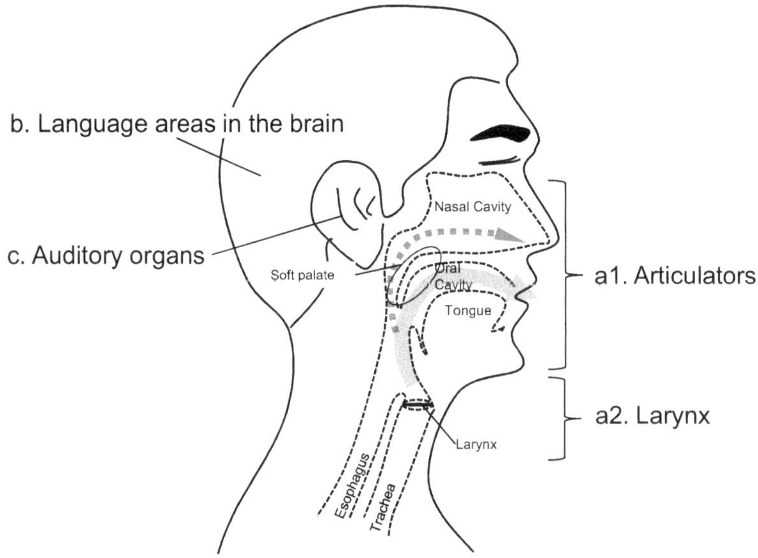

Fig. 9.1 Categories of causes of speech and language impairment

9.1.1.2 Methods for Assisting Voice Production and Electrolarynx

The electrolarynx is currently described as a technology for practical use. Patients who have their larynx removed due to cancer of the larynx also lose their vocal cords and breathe through tracheostomy in the throat. In this case, the route from the mouth to the lungs is blocked to prevent food from entering the respiratory tract, and the respiratory tract and esophagus are kept separate. Thus, they lose the source of the original voice sound and the path of the expiratory flow for vocalization, so they cannot produce voices, including whispers.

Typical alternative phonation methods include esophageal speech, tracheoesophageal speech (T-E shunt method), and the electrolarynx. Figure 9.2 shows a schematic illustration of esophageal speech and the electrolarynx.

During esophageal phonation, the pharyngoesophageal sphincter vibrates as if burping, and this sound becomes the source of vocal sounds. In the T-E shunt method, small airflow shunts are opened between the trachea and esophagus so that when the tracheostomy is blocked by a finger, exhaled air flows into the esophagus, and a part of the esophagus vibrates.

It takes a lot of practice to learn esophageal vocalization, and various organizations for laryngectomized patients hold vocal training classes. These activities contribute not only to speech rehabilitation but also to mental support and quality of life improvement before and after surgery [1]. However, one drawback of this method is that the necessary training, which is both demanding and exhausting, makes it particularly difficult, if not impossible, for the elderly to master.

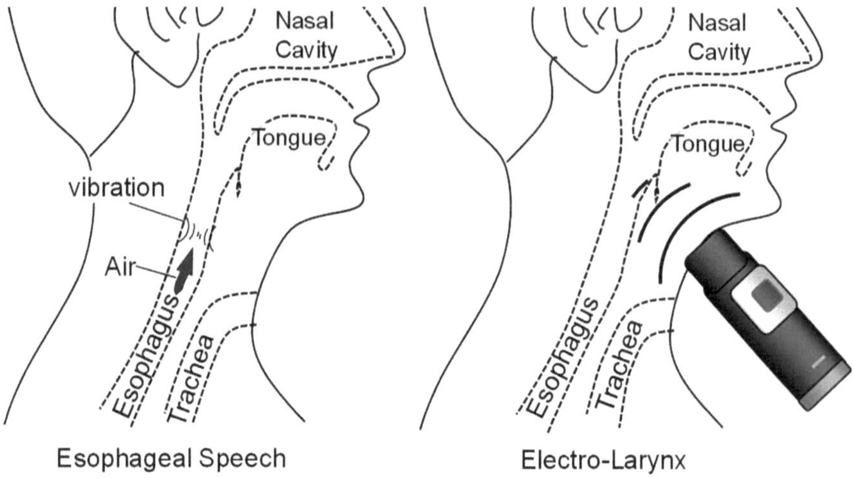

Fig. 9.2 Illustrations of esophageal speech method and electrolarynx

An electric larynx is a device in which an electrically driven vibrator is pressed under the jaw to deliver vibrating sound as a vocal source into the vocal tract, enabling speech. An advantage of this method is that it is easy to learn. Further, because there is no need to exhale, it is possible to vocalize as much as the user wants without worrying about breathing. The drawback is that the sound quality often sounds like a buzzer. Moreover, as some vibration sounds leak from the vocal tract, they may interfere with the listener. There is also the inconvenience of using the device in the hand. Although there are advantages and disadvantages in terms of sound quality, ease of training, and ease of hygiene maintenance, there are many users of the electrolarynx because of its noninvasiveness and ease of learning, and the percentage of users is increasing [2].

There have been several studies and developments to compensate for the shortcomings of the electric larynx, and this technology has been progressing.

Uemi et al. designed an electrolarynx that allowed pitch control [3]. Hashiba et al. are also contributing to the production of an electric larynx with natural speech fluctuations [4] and the development of a wearable electric larynx [5]. Takeuchi et al. attempted to improve the shortcomings of sound quality and volume by combining multiple vibrators [6].

9.1.1.3 Text to Speech (TTS) and Augmentative and Alternative Communication (AAC)

Speech disorders can be caused by partial impairment of the vocal and articular organs, but they are often caused by central disorders or diseases of the muscles and nervous system throughout the body. Augmented alternative communication (AAC) and voice output communication assistants (VOCAs), which enable communication by means of tools and devices such as picture boards, character boards, switch devices, and voice output devices, are used according to the patient's condition.

Some VOCAs already available are those in which a registered voice is output when a button on which a picture symbol is drawn is pressed and those in which an arbitrary sentence or word entered with a letter key can be output by text-to-speech (TTS) synthesis. Recently, many of them have been released as tablet applications, and some have additional functions such as e-mail, in addition to voice output.

Augmentative and alternative communication devices, which combine software with personalized switch controllers, are used in patients with more severe musculoskeletal conditions. In amyotrophic lateral sclerosis (ALS), for example, as the disease progresses through initial symptoms, such as weakness of the hands and feet, the muscles of the vocal, articular, and respiratory organs gradually lose their ability to speak. When the patient becomes serious, it becomes difficult to use the normal key input because of the muscle weakness of the whole body, and special input devices are required. In this case, it is possible to operate a PC or tablet terminal with minute movements of the body or eye and output speech. In addition to gaze input, input by a scan interface in which a cursor automatically scans a character list arranged in a matrix and selects a character according to the timing of pressing one switch is often used as an input method. There is also an input method in which the selection is made using biological information, such as brain waves and cerebral blood flow. Switches are required to detect even slight forces or movements, such as blinking or exhalation. In addition to the electrical contact method, electrified, exhaled (intake), photoelectric, piezoelectric, and myoelectric switches have been developed. The selection and setting of these devices require knowledge and expertise in consideration of changes due to the progression of the disease.

The speech devices described above usually output speech using TTS synthesis technology. In recent years, some TTS synthesizers have used AI technology to reproduce the voices of patients. These AI speech synthesis methods are limited in the available languages and require a substantial amount of voice recording to build a database, which could be expensive. More recently, speech synthesis systems that can output sound similar to a person's voice from recordings of several minutes or tens of seconds have emerged, and future developments are expected. In the case of diseases such as laryngectomy and ALS, it is important to record and store one's own voice before losing it, since it is predictable that one will lose voice due to surgery or disease progression.

On the other hand, it is important to note that the expression "similar voice" implies that there are features that do not equal one's own voice. In many cases, the voice synthesized from a limited database does not reproduce the intonation or the way of speaking like the person, even if the tone sounds like the person.

An example of preserving and using patients' voices is the "MyVoice" tool included in the Japanese AAC software HeartyLadder [7]. The software attempted to use as much of the patient's recorded voice as possible. Although the fluency of continuous speech is inferior to that of commercially available TTS voice, it is preferred for emotional communication with family and friends because it outputs almost all raw speech, such as words actually recorded by the patient. The software registers each word with the support of the medical worker. In daily life, when the disease weakens speech muscles, the patient chooses what words to register and how to speak them in cooperation with family and medical personnel and increases the number of recorded words. In some cases, increasing the number of recorded words may be pleasurable for the patients themselves. The voice output from the system also provides others with a sense of the patient's personality. Such efforts to preserve the patient's voice contribute to the mental support of not only the patient but also the family members who support the patient. Thus, the author believes that it is important to note that there are cases in which the patient's own voice is desirable, even if it is not fluent.

9.1.2 Research and Development for Articulation Disorders and Their Positioning

9.1.2.1 Attempt to Complement Articulation Function with Formant Control

This section introduces a system that focuses on articulation disorders. Articulation disorders occur when the vocal tract converts the original sound produced by vocal cords into sounds that can be heard as spoken words. Because many parts of the organs are associated, the causes and severity vary. The causes of articulation disorders can be broadly classified into motor, organic, functional, and auditory, and the support methods differ for each. In dentistry and medicine, surgical treatment and aid are used to improve speech sound quality. In rehabilitation, some approaches are used to visualize a patient's voice to evaluate articulation problems and guide correct pronunciation. If treatment and rehabilitation are not effective, some kind of equipment or tools are used; however, currently, there are few practical devices that focus on articulation disorders, and in most cases, speech synthesis and writing are used.

As a speech generator that focuses on the articulation function, the authors proposed a speech-generating device that replaces the movement of the human articulation system with the position and movement of the finger (Fig. 9.3). The device instantly outputs a voice corresponding to the position of a finger or pen on an operating board surface arranged with the first formant (F1) and second formant (F2) as coordinate axes by formant speech synthesis (Fig. 9.4) [8]. This device is intended to be able to express rhythm, pauses, and intonation as if it were a part of the body by changing the sound according to the position in a nonstep manner, providing immediacy like a musical instrument. A speech-generating application using this method was released for iOS in 2013 under the name "Yubide Hanasou," which means "Let's talk with a finger" in Japanese [9].

The positions of the vowels placed by F1 and F2 were closely related to the position of the tongue when vowels were produced. The positions of the highest parts of the tongue during the generation of vowels are analogous to the positional

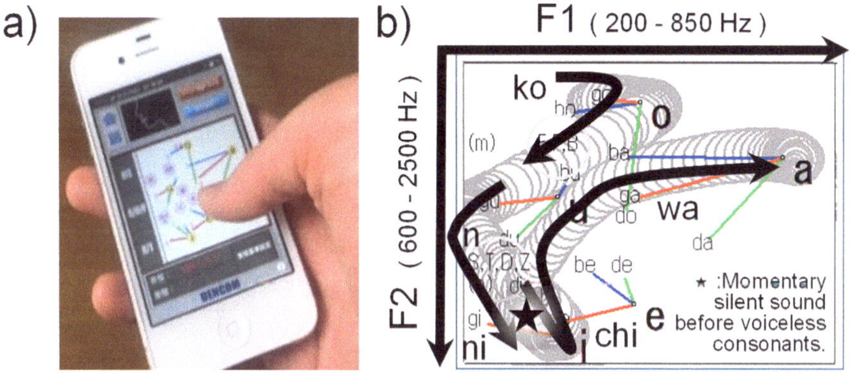

Fig. 9.3 (**a**) Speech generating application "Yubide-Hanasou", (**b**) Example of finger trajectory to generate "Konnichiwa" (Japanese for Hello)

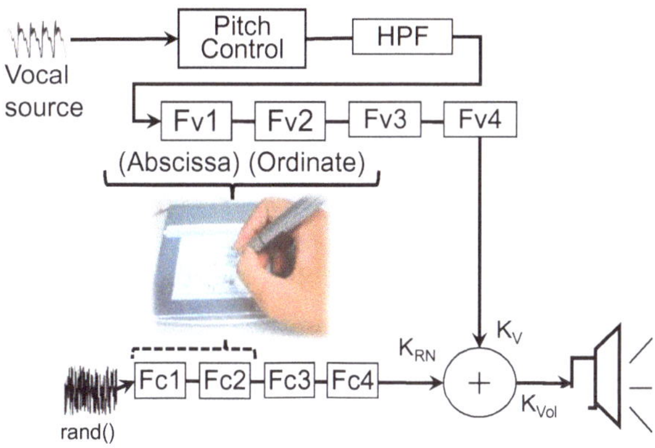

Fig. 9.4 Block diagram of speech generating system controlled by F1–F2 interface

relationships of the vowels in the operation panel (Fig. 9.5). Maintaining this continuous relationship between phonemic elements is also important for replacing the human articulation mechanism.

In this system, because the control of phonology and prosody is independent, the pitch and intonation of voice can be controlled independently of phonology by adding an interface. For example, voice pitch can be assigned to the tilt of a smartphone or a pressure sensor to control inflection in real time. In experiments in which the pressure of a tracing finger or pen tablet was assigned to the pitch of the original sound, it was demonstrated that it is possible to easily generate a vowel voice with emotions and a sound of laughter composed of each vowel. It was also possible to sing songs by manipulating phonology with a pen in the left hand and playing keyboard instruments connected via MIDI in the right hand (Fig. 9.6) [10]. Thus, the ability to control both phonology and the source sound in real time greatly increases the degree of flexibility compared with text-to-speech synthesis, and it is possible to produce a sense of enjoyment.

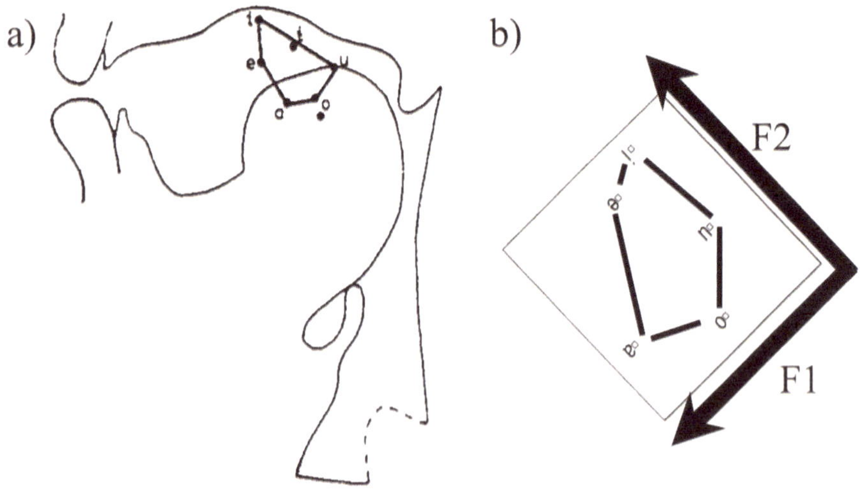

Fig. 9.5 (**a**) The highest points of the tongue of the vowels (by G. Fant [12]), (**b**) control plane of the software

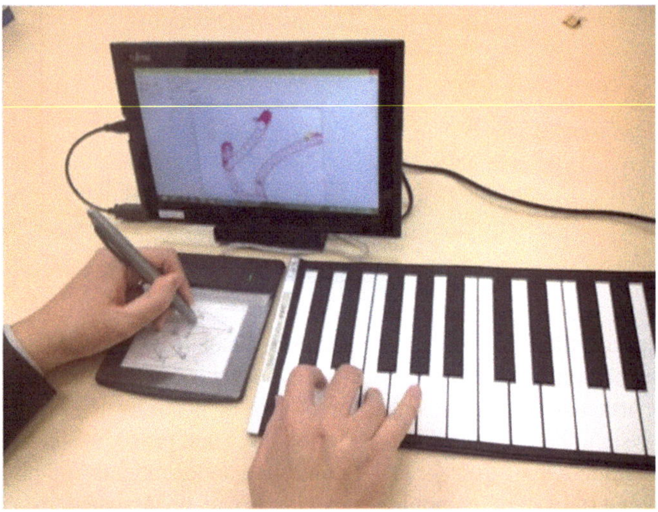

Fig. 9.6 A System that enables singing with phonological control on an F1–F2 interface

By extending this method, if only articulation is impaired, it would be possible to generate articulated speech in real time while maintaining voice qualities by adding inputs besides the voice as the speaker is speaking. The authors have developed a prototype device that adds phonological features in real time by using the voice of a user with an articulation disorder in which the voicing function remains and demonstrated its potential [11]. Figure 9.7 shows a schematic of a prototype mobile device equipped with functions such as voice conversion, input/output, and power

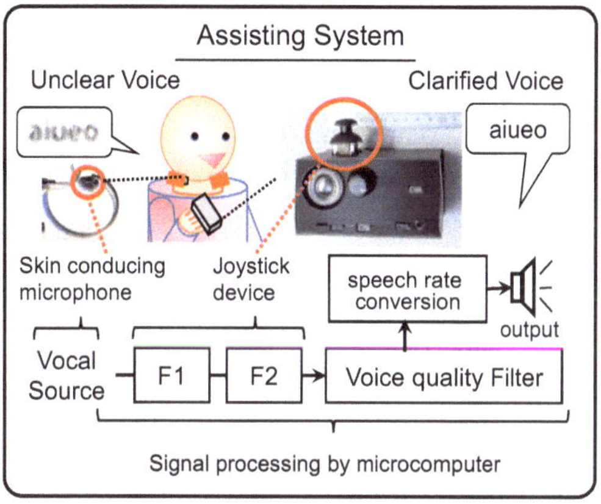

Fig. 9.7 An outline of a speech-assisting system using a speaker's voice as a sound source

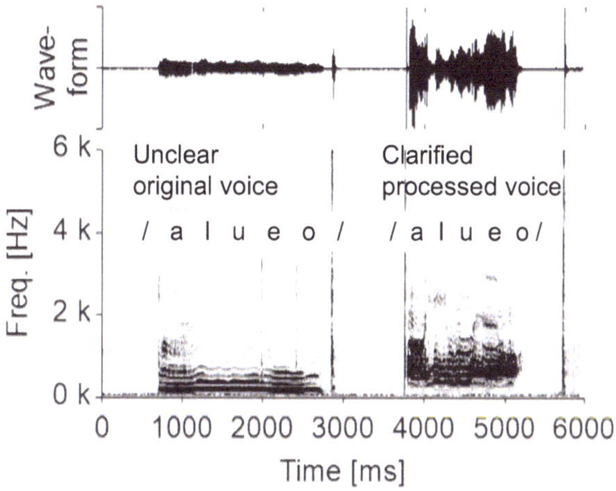

Fig. 9.8 Wave-forms and spectrograms of the original unclear voice and the clarified voice

supply. The source sound was acquired from a skin conduction microphone attached to the user's neck. The voice signal is subjected to a filtering process for characterizing F1 and F2 and correcting voice quality, including individual characteristics, so that prosody and other characteristics are maintained and the articulatory voice is corrected. An analysis of the speaker's voice recorded during the experiment and the voice from the device is shown in Fig. 9.8. In the spectrogram of the voice converted from the original speaker voice with little spectral change, a formant change due to the F1-F2 characterization can be observed.

Although this method shows a certain possibility for correcting articulation, there are still some difficulties. The sound quality is not stable in some cases, depending on the position and contact of the skin conduction microphone, and it is difficult to operate the phonology accurately by hand. Another difficulty is that the clarity of words is not high because only formant movements produce consonant-like sounds.

There are various other approaches to improve or clarify the voice quality of speech in articulation disorders that are expected to develop in the future. It is important to note that many nonverbal information other than phonology remain in the voice spoken by the speech organs in patients with articulation disorders, and they have important roles. This should be aimed at the development of a system capable of outputting clear speech while keeping the nonverbal information contained in the prosody and the manner of each speaker, not only the verbal content.

9.1.2.2 Attempt to Assist Voice Feedback by Speech-Rate Conversion

Another approach to support articulation disorders is rehabilitation. In this section, research on applications for assisting speech rehabilitation using speech-rate conversion is introduced.

Patients with articulation disorders due to diseases of the cerebral and neurological systems are often treated with rehabilitation by a speech-language-hearing therapist (ST) to relearn articulatory movements. Articulatory movement is the appropriate movement of speech organs such as the tongue and lips. The authors studied the voices of patients in the cerebral and nervous systems with the cooperation of speech therapists. During the study, there were many cases in which there appeared to be a disproportion between the speed at which the speaker intended to speak and the accuracy of articulation that could be achieved. That is, there is a tradeoff between moving the articulator at the right position and trajectory and moving it at high speed.

Slowing the speech speed according to the recovery level of the patient makes it easier to move the articular organs in the appropriate position and trajectory, and it is suggested that inducing a slow speech speed would help the training process. In speech therapist training, there are various ways to control the speed. However, there is a difference between the slow speech of a normal speaker and that of a patient with slow articulation. Slowly spoken voices of normal speakers usually produce a voice in which vowels are elongated without slowing down the articulation of consonants. In contrast, a voice spoken with slow articulation also slows the articulation of the consonant. Such speech sounds are unnatural, even if the position and trajectory of the articulation organs are correct. If the speed is increased to eliminate this unnaturalness, the accuracy of the position and trajectory of the articulation organs will become insufficient.

The authors have been developing applications based on tablet devices, focusing on the fact that the unnaturalness observed in a patient's slow speech is similar to the unnaturalness of a voice slowed by speech-rate conversion. The application aims for two effects with two patterns of speech-rate conversion (Fig. 9.9).

The first function is to reduce the speed of speech to be presented as a practice model using speech-rate conversion. The speech reduced in speed presented here contains unnaturalness peculiar to speech reduction by speech-rate conversion. By imitating a slow voice that contains unnaturalness, the patient aims to train the articulator to move in the correct position and trajectory, even at slow speeds that contain unnaturalness.

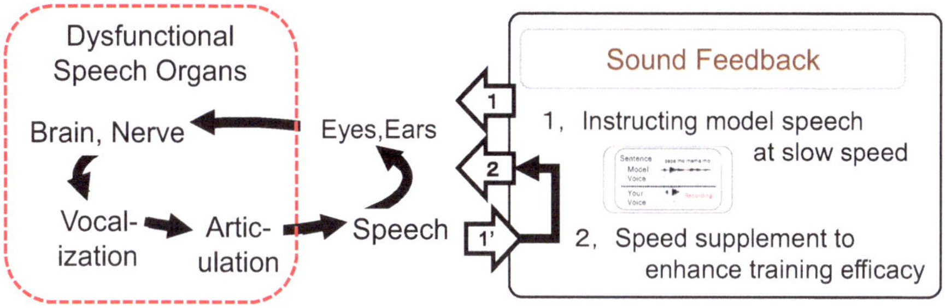

Fig. 9.9 Concept of voice feedback assisting with speed conversion technology

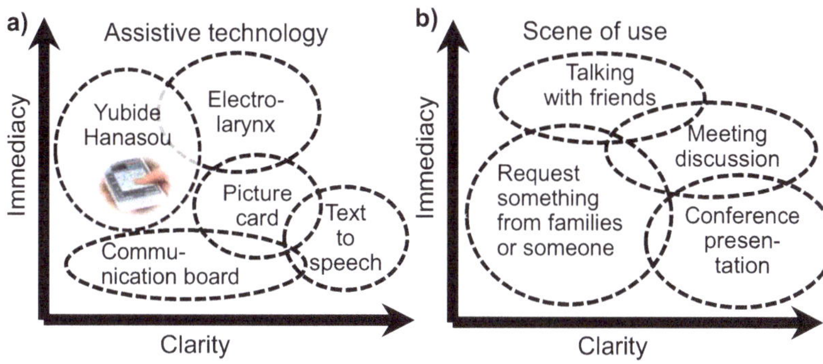

Fig. 9.10 (**a**) Supported level of immediacies and clarities of each method of communication aid; (**b**) needed level of immediacies and clarities for each communication scene

The second function is to speed up the patient's slow speech by speech-rate conversion and provide feedback to the patient. The patient's voice is converted to a speed as fast as the model voice, which eliminates unnaturalness caused by slow voice. By listening to this speech, the patient may be aware that the voice is satisfactory if correct articulation is achieved, even if the voice is slow.

An application that provides supplementary functions, such as waveform display, in addition to these speed-changing functions, is currently being tested and analyzed.

9.1.3 Positioning of Each Method

9.1.3.1 Immediacy and Clarity

Speech support technology has been previously described. It should be noted that target needs differ depending on the type and degree of each disability.

For example, when focusing on immediacy and clarity, the positioning of the aforementioned communication support methods is schematically shown in

Fig. 9.10a. Similarly, Fig. 9.10b conceptually illustrates the immediacy and clarity required for some of the assumed situations.

Depending on the situation in which the device is used, there are different needs to be prioritized, and the appropriate assisting devices differ accordingly. For example, in speeches or presentations at conferences, which can be prepared in advance, speech synthesis is an appropriate method because it is required to deliver as clearly as possible. However, in the case of small talk with several people, immediacy is extremely important because the speaker or topic changes one after another. If there is even a 5-s pause, another speaker will immediately interrupt and change the subject, and it is impossible to join the conversation without speaking before that. An electric larynx can produce a voice when pushing a button, so it can be used in situations where both immediacy and clarity are required. However, this is difficult in patients with articulation disorders.

If the topic of conversation is limited and the listener is close to the speaker or if it is possible to confirm what is being said interactively, it is possible to communicate what is being said by a situation or physical movement. In such cases, immediacy, rather than clarity, is required. People with arthritic disorders often prefer to speak in their own voice, even when their speech is unclear. This may be because of the importance of immediacy and other verbal and nonverbal information.

9.1.3.2 Speech Information Other than Language

Patients with cerebral and nervous system disorders may have difficulty recognizing letters, typing, or expressing clear semantic information. In such cases, the intention may be communicated through a unique gesture or vocal expression that can only be understood by the family member and the parent. As in the F1-F2 articulation simulation system like "Yubide Hanasou" described above, if the degrees of flexibility are used appropriately, such as the change in the middle sound between vowels and the change in the pitch of the voice, it may be possible to use it freely without being bound by "language."

Handling paralanguage and nonverbal information in text-to-speech synthesis and support by the electrolarynx has long been a major issue. It is often said that voice-assisted devices do not convey emotions; however, it is questionable whether emotions are what users really want. Mori et al. pointed out the positioning of both automatic involuntary and messaging aspects of emotional expression [13]. The information users probably want may not be an expression of an involuntary state of mind but rather paraverbal or similar information with the active message aspect of emotions. The issue of what the physical quantity of such information is and what kind of input operation it should be connected to has not yet been solved.

In relation to nonverbal information, there are also issues regarding the expression of individuality. In continuous speech synthesis using one's own voice, there are often comments such as, "It's my voice, but it's not my voice." Even if a recording is made by the same person, the voice is completely different depending on the time and place of recording and the beginning and end of the recording. These comments suggest that individuality includes something different from voice quality and that voice quality varies widely, even within an individual.

The topics described in this chapter on support for speech disorders are obviously only part of them. However, it would be appreciated if some of the examples and perspectives described in this chapter could help highly skilled readers apply these to new assistive technologies.

9.2 Assisting Deaf and Hard of Hearing (DHH): Information Acquisition Support

9.2.1 Introduction

The World Health Organization (WHO) reported that around 1.5 billion people worldwide have some degree of hearing loss, and over 430 million are affected by hearing impairments [14]. Moreover, about one in four people globally—approximately 2.5 billion—is expected to experience some hearing loss, with more than 700 million likely to have a moderate or more severe level of hearing loss [14]. The global burden of hearing loss is unevenly distributed, with low- and middle-income countries taking on a disproportionate amount. Common causes of hearing loss worldwide include chronic otitis media, noise-induced hearing loss, age-related loss, and congenital conditions [15]. The leading causes of acquired hearing loss include age-related (presbycusis) and noise-induced hearing loss [16, 17].

As a specific example, Japan had approximately 379,000 people with hearing or speech impairment as of 2022 [18]. Similar to visual impairment, the age distribution shows a predominance of older adults, with approximately 9000 people under the age of 20 years, 87,000 people aged 20–64 years, and 283,000 people aged 65 years and over [5]. The causes of hearing impairment in Japan involve complex interactions between genetic and environmental factors. More than 50% of all congenital hearing disorders are associated with 80 or 100 different genes related to hearing loss [19], highlighting the significant genetic component of hearing impairment. However, the most common cause of hearing impairment in those under 20 years of age remains unknown (65%), followed by cochlear nerve canal/inner ear canal stenosis (21%) and cochlear malformation (7%) [20]. Among adults aged 20 years or older, sudden hearing loss emerges as the most common cause (49–66%), followed by unknown causes (8.6–32%) and Meniere's disease (5.5–13%) [21]. The causes of hearing loss show distinct age-related patterns, with Meniere's disease occurring most frequently in people aged in their 40s–70s, while mumps hearing loss and acoustic trauma occur most frequently in people aged in their 20s–30s [21]. These patterns suggest different risk factors and exposure patterns across the lifespan. Moreover, hearing loss is recognized as a risk factor for dementia, and early detection, along with appropriate interventions for acquired hearing loss, is crucial for dementia prevention [22, 23].

Comprehensive support systems have evolved over centuries, with deaf education representing one of the earliest forms of systematic disability support, spanning over 400 years since Pedro Ponce de Leon's pioneering work in sixteenth-century Spain [24]. Formal deaf education began with Abbe Charles-Michel de l'Epee's establishment of the first public school for the deaf in Paris (1760), pioneering sign language instruction [24]. Modern legal frameworks emphasize accessibility rights through the Americans with Disabilities Act (1990), European Accessibility Act (2019), and the UN Convention on the Rights of Persons with Disabilities (2006), which recognized sign languages as full languages. As an eastern country, Japan's first deaf school was established in 1878 [25]. Key legislation includes the Act on the Welfare of Persons with Disabilities (1949), Sign Language Recognition Law (2011), officially recognizing Japanese Sign Language, and the Law for Eliminating Discrimination against Persons with Disabilities (2016) [18]. Modern support relies on technological solutions, including real-time captioning and digital accessibility standards such as WCAG 2.1 [26, 27].

Building on this rich historical background and modern accessibility frameworks, this chapter focuses on information support systems for people with hearing impairments. The chapter will examine recent technological innovations in communication support and their incorporation into holistically designed frameworks that honor individual communication preferences and deaf cultural values.

9.2.2 Hearing Impaired Status

Hearing impairments can be categorized as deaf or hard of hearing (DHH) based on international standards. The former indicates a state of total hearing loss (HL), with most cases having a hearing level of 90–100 dB or higher. The latter pertains to a reduced hearing level (>20 dB HL). Various classifications of hearing loss exist, but generally, a hearing loss of 20–40 dB in the better ear is considered mild (or Grade 1), 40–60 dB as moderate (or Grade 2), 60–80 to 90 dB as severe (or Grade 3), and 80–90 dB or higher as profound hearing loss (or Grade 4) [28, 29]. In studies supporting people with DHH, most focus on those with severe hearing loss or higher grades. Note that this criterion only refers to hearing level, and individuals' communication methods vary; some use sign language, some rely on spoken communication, and others use written communication.

9.2.3 Information Assurance

Information assurance for the hearing impaired can be divided into two main categories: hearing assistance for the hard of hearing and the conversion and presentation of sound information into visual information for people who are deaf or hard of hearing.

9.2.3.1 Hearing Aid and Cochlear Implant

The first step in helping those who are hard of hearing and deaf is using hearing aids and cochlear implants to enhance their hearing [30].

For hearing aids, pocket and in-ear options are available, primarily from manufacturers such as Rion, Resound, Panasonic, and Philips. Cochlear implants consist of two parts: internally implanted components within the inner ear and external devices, including a transmitter coil, such as those produced by Cochlear and MED-EL. In these technologies, it is crucial not only to amplify sounds but also to suppress noise and enhance desired sounds [31]. Specifically, Levitt mentions that random noise, competing voices, and significant room reverberation should be suppressed. Alongside spectrum-based noise reduction and source direction-based methods, adaptive filtering techniques have been studied for many years as solutions to these issues, leading to ongoing improvements in audibility that are constantly being made [32–34]. As the design of hearing aids improves, similar to eyewear, some deaf communities have started to adopt fashion-forward approaches, transforming reported trends in some deaf communities [35]. What was once considered a stigma has been transformed into a fashion statement.

When using these hearing devices, it is important to fine-tune amplification settings to match each person's hearing abilities. During the COVID-19 pandemic, mobile apps for diagnosing hearing loss have become more widespread [36], while teleaudiology, a method enabling remote and accurate hearing assessments by specialists, has been studied [37].

Some hearing aids and cochlear implants feature wireless speech transmission, including hearing loops, frequency modulation (FM) hearing systems, and digital assistive listening devices such as Roger [38–40]. Hearing loops utilize electrical wires installed on the floor or ceiling to magnetize speech signals, which are then received by devices with a telecoil integrated into hearing aids and cochlear implants. Meanwhile, FM systems and digital assistive listening systems are portable and have simpler sound collection units that connect directly to hearing devices.

9.2.3.2 Real-Time Captioning

Written summaries and real-time captioning are common methods of information access for people with DHH. In Japan, NHK broadcaster began subtitling live news programs using speech recognition in 2000 [41], and the *respeak* method has enabled subtitling of shows other than news programs. The *respeak* method enhances recognition rates and adds to the content by having the subtitle caster repeat the content [42]; many programs now support subtitle broadcasting. At academic conferences and lectures, text is often manually inputted into a computer and displayed on a screen. Collaborative input is frequently performed by two people [43] in Japan, and crowdsourcing is used to generate subtitles [44], mainly in English-speaking countries. Currently, speech recognition is used in more cases, but it requires a proofreader, depending on the environment where the voice is recorded.

Remote information assurance support involves transmitting voice to a remote location via the Internet and sending text information back to a mobile device from that location. Recently, the adoption of remote systems has surged due to the swift implementation of measures to prevent COVID-19 infections. While these systems primarily function as unidirectional real-time subtitles, there is an increasing need for interactivity. For example, enabling students with hearing impairments to ask questions directly to faculty members is a priority. Ongoing research and development aim to enhance these capabilities [45].

9.2.4 Communication Support

9.2.4.1 Use of Speech Recognition and Text-to-Speech Applications

Now that advanced speech recognition technology is widely available, there has been rapid growth in smartphone applications designed to assist the hearing impaired. Notable examples include *UDTalk* [46] and *KoeTra* [47]. These apps convert spoken words from a person with normal hearing into text using speech recognition, while text input from a person with hearing impairment who has difficulty speaking can be outputted audibly through text to speech. Similar technology has also been developed for applications that translate into foreign languages [48].

Research has examined how such subtitles are presented. For example, when scrolling subtitles from bottom to top, hearing-impaired participants did not always follow the subtitles as they appeared [49]. Additionally, while participants without hearing impairments stopped their gaze at the ",", those with impairments preferred the sentence with a line break instead of the ",."

9.2.4.2 Intercommunication Between Speech, Writing, and Sign Language

Congenitally profoundly deaf individuals whose native language is sign language and who have never acquired a spoken language may struggle to understand written words. Although the age for cochlear implant surgery in children has been brought forward for better spoken language development [50], the importance of sign language as a means of communication for the DHH people remains unquestioned. Research has been conducted on sign language interpretation through image recognition and computer graphics, with best practices documented for telecommunications and other delays [51].

9.2.5 *Various Supports for the DHH*

The technologies mentioned above are used to assist the social activities of hearing-impaired individuals. Particularly, this section discusses actual examples in educational settings and sports environments.

9.2.5.1 Supports in Education Sites

A growing number of case studies have examined e-learning systems for people with various disabilities, especially cognitive or learning disabilities [52, 53]. Particularly, Farhan et al. designed a Web-based e-learning interface that allows students with and without hearing and visual impairments to collaborate in inclusive educational settings [54]. In addition to visual supports such as text and graphics, this system could simultaneously display sign language animations, and users were highly satisfied with using the system regardless of their disability status.

Nonetheless, verifying the effectiveness of assistive technology for individuals with hearing impairments in educational settings still requires improvement. Bell et al. reviewed practical studies and found few that offer promising, evidence-based data on how hearing assistive technology impacts educational success [55]. Consequently, future research should explore ways to better utilize assistive technology to enhance educational outcomes for individuals with hearing impairments and gather scientific evidence of its effectiveness.

9.2.5.2 Participating Sports for Deaf

Support for social activities for the hearing impaired exists, similar to support for the visually impaired. Specifically, assistance in sports for the hearing impaired can be categorized into two main types: viewing and competing.

In the former category, a study was conducted around 1980 on a TV captioning system for the hearing impaired, with subtitling of sports programs used as an example of an application [56]. As an example of sign language translation, Othman et al. created *SportsSign*, a Web tool that displays sports news in sign language with avatars [57]. Uchida et al. developed a similar system that generates Japanese sign language animations in real time alongside sports situations [58]. Regarding a system for presenting tactile modalities, Shibasaki et al. reported a system that transmits tap dancers' movements on stage to hearing-impaired audience members using vibrotactile sensation [59].

The latter includes systems that support the implementation of competitions and the development of motor skills. Peñeñory et al. reviewed studies on psychomotor skills in children with hearing impairment and categorized them into two groups: support for coordination, balance, and posture related to fundamental motor skills and support for spatial, temporal, and rhythmic perception related to perceptual motor skills [60]. Jaijun et al. found that integrating mobile Internet technology into physical education courses enhanced student persistence and self-efficacy by improving teacher-student interactions [61]. Such skill development extends beyond athletics; for example, Elvitigala et al. created *SwimSight*, a system that visually displays swimming times and other related information [62], and Shitara et al. developed *HaptStarter*, a haptic start display to ensure a simultaneous start sign for DHH sprinters [63].

9.2.6 Conclusion

Modern information assurance for DHH individuals operates through two primary mechanisms: hearing enhancement for those with residual hearing and converting auditory information into visual formats for those with profound hearing loss. Hearing aids and cochlear implants are the core technologies, featuring advanced options such as noise suppression, directional microphones, and wireless connectivity via hearing loops, FM systems, and digital assistive listening devices. The COVID-19 pandemic sped up the use of teleaudiology and smartphone-based hearing assessment apps, showing the potential for remote diagnostic and treatment options.

Real-time captioning has become an essential accessibility tool, with uses ranging from broadcast television subtitles using speech recognition technology to collaborative manual input systems for academic conferences. The respeak method, developed in Japan, improves recognition accuracy by having trained operators repeat content for speech recognition systems. Remote captioning services have grown quickly, though challenges still exist in achieving two-way communication and maintaining accuracy across different acoustic settings.

Communication support applications leverage advanced speech recognition and text-to-speech technologies to facilitate interactions between hearing and DHH individuals. Applications such as UDTalk and KoeTra provide real-time conversion between spoken language and text, while ongoing research explores intercommunication systems that feature sign language recognition and generation capabilities.

Educational applications show the potential for inclusive learning environments, with Web-based platforms supporting collaborative learning among students with and without hearing impairments. However, systematic evaluation of educational outcomes remains limited, highlighting the need for evidence-based research on assistive technology effectiveness. Similarly, support for sports participation includes both spectator accessibility through captioned broadcasts and sign language interpretation, as well as competitive systems that improve motor skills and provide real-time performance feedback.

References

1. Geng, J., Xi, S., Wu, P.: A qualitative study on experiences of patients with Esophageal speech training after total laryngectomy. Yangtze Medicine. **5**, 179–193 (2021). https://doi.org/10.4236/ym.2021.53018
2. Kanazawa, S., Yoshino, K., Fujii, T., et al.: Voice rehabilitation, alaryngeal communication and swallowing function after total laryngectomy (in Japanese). J. Jpn. Soc. Head Neck Surg. **22**, 303–310 (2012). https://doi.org/10.5106/jjshns.22.303
3. Uemi, N., Ifukube, T., Takahashi, M., Matsushima, J.: Design of a new electrolarynx having a pitch control function. In: 3rd IEEE International Workshop on Robot and Human Communication, 1994. RO-MAN '94 Nagoya, Proceedings, pp. 198–203 (1994)
4. Commercialization of the New Electro-larynx having Natural Fluctuation of Voice (in Japanese). https://www.hro.or.jp/upload/27294/23.pdf
5. Hashiba, M., Sugai, Y., Izumi, T., et al.: Development of a wearable electro-larynx for laryngectomees and its evaluation. In: 29th Annual International Conference of the IEEE Engineering in Medicine and Biology Society, 2007. EMBS 2007, pp. 5267–5270 (2007)
6. Takeuchi, M., Ahn, J., Lee, K., et al.: Hands-free wearable electrolarynx using linear predictive coding residual waves and listening evaluation. Adv. Biomed. Eng. **11**, 68–75 (2022). https://doi.org/10.14326/abe.11.68
7. Kawahara, S., Homma, M., Yoshimura, T., Arai, T.: MyVoice: rescuing voices of ALS patients. Acoust. Sci. Technol. **37**, 202–210 (2016). https://doi.org/10.1250/ast.37.202
8. Yabu, K., Ifukube, T., Aomura, S.: A speech synthesis method using a pointing device: as a speaking aid for speech disorders. Jpn. Acad. Health Sci. **12**, 49–57 (2009). https://doi.org/10.24531/jhsaiih.12.1_49
9. Hashiba, M., Yabu, K., Takase, M., Sugai, Y., Ifukube, T.: Development of a real-time speech synthesis application software for smartphone controlled by finger positions and movements. (in Japanese). In: Proceedings of the Human Interface Symposium 2013:ROMBUNNO.2501D (2013)
10. Yabu, K., Ifukube, T., Aomura, S.: Expression of non-verbal information for a speech synthesis method using a pointing device: as an emotional expression aid during communication. Jpn. Acad. Health Sci. **12**, 117–124 (2009). https://doi.org/10.24531/jhsaiih.12.2_117
11. Yabu, K., Tanaka, T., Ifukube, T.: A prototype of wearable real-time speech processing device for assisting articulation disorders. Rep. Spring Meet. Acoust. Soc. Jpn. **2025**, 801–802 (2025)
12. Fant, G.: Acoustic Theory of Speech Production, pp. 111–112. Walter de Gruyter (1970)
13. Mori, H., Nakamura, M.: Interpretation of the concept of emotion in speech studies. (in Japanese). J. Acoust. Soc. Jpn. **71**, 461–467 (2015). https://doi.org/10.20697/jasj.71.9_461
14. World Health Organization, World report on hearing, https://www.who.int/publications/i/item/9789240020481 (2021)
15. Wilson, B.S., Tucci, D.L., Merson, M.H., O'Donoghue, G.M.: Lancet. **390**(10111), 2503 (2017)
16. Dobie, R.A.: Ear Hear. **29**(4), 565 (2008)
17. Haile, L.M., Orji, A.U., Reavis, K.M., Briant, P.S., Lucas, K.M., Alahdab, F., Bärnighausen, T. W., Bell, A.W., Cao, C., Dai, X., et al.: Ear Hear. **45**(1), 257 (2024)
18. Ministry of Health, Labour and Welfare, Japan. https://www.mhlw.go.jp/content/11704000/000955880.pdf (2022)
19. Shimada, A.: Shikoku Acta Medica. **71**(5–6), 111 (2015)
20. Kashio, A., Koyama, H., ichi Nishimura, S., Doi, K., Nakagawa, T., Iwasaki, S., Ito, K., Yamasoba, T.: Audiol. Jpn. **64**(5), 507 (2021)
21. Koyama, H., Kashio, A., ichi Nishimura, S., Iwasaki, S., Doi, K., Nakagawa, T., Ito, K.: Audiol. Jpn. **64**(5), 501 (2021)
22. Livingston, G., Sommerlad, A., Orgeta, V., Costafreda, S.G., Huntley, J., Ames, D., Ballard, C., Banerjee, S., Burns, A., Cohen-Mansfield, J., et al.: Lancet. **390**(10113), 2673 (2017)

23. Livingston, G., Huntley, J., Sommerlad, A., Ames, D., Ballard, C., Banerjee, S., Brayne, C., Burns, A., Cohen-Mansfield, J., Cooper, C., et al.: Lancet. **396**(10248), 413 (2020)
24. Lane, H.: When the Mind Hears: A History of the Deaf. Vintage (1989)
25. Nakamura, K.: Deaf in Japan: Signing and the Politics of Identity. Cornell University Press (2006)
26. Web content accessibility guidelines (wcag) 2.1.. https://www.w3.org/TR/WCAG21/
27. Alsalamah, A.: Am. Ann. Deaf. **165**(1), 114 (2020)
28. Sato, M., Matsunaga, T., Kanzaki, J., Ogawa, K., Inoue, Y., Houya, N.: Nippon Jibiinkoka Gakkai Kaiho. **104**(3), 192 (2001)
29. Olusanya, B.O., Davis, A.C., Hoffman, H.J.: Bull. World Health Organ. **97**(10), 725 (2019)
30. Haumann, S., Hohmann, V., Meis, M., Herzke, T., Lenarz, T., Büchner, A.: Audiol. Res. **2**(1), e12 (2012)
31. Rudner, M., Rönnberg, J., Lunner, T.: J. Am. Acad. Audiol. **22**(03), 156 (2011)
32. Levitt, H.: J. Rehabil. Res. Dev. **38**(1), 111 (2001)
33. Mauger, S.J., Arora, K., Dawson, P.W.: J. Neural Eng. **9**(6), 065007 (2012)
34. Bentler, R.A.: J. Am. Acad. Audiol. **16**(07), 473 (2005)
35. Profita, H.P., Stangl, A., Matuszewska, L., Sky, S., Kushalnagar, R., Kane, S.K.: ACM Trans. Access. Comput. **11**(3), 1 (2018)
36. Irace, A.L., Sharma, R.K., Reed, N.S., Golub, J.S.: J. Am. Geriatr. Soc. **69**(2), 307 (2021)
37. Kim, J., Jeon, S., Kim, D., Shin, Y.: J. Audiol. Otol. **25**(1), 1 (2021)
38. Myers, D.G.: Perspect. Psychol. Sci. **14**(1), 29 (2019)
39. Schaeffer, C.: Public Libr. Q. **32**(4), 319 (2013)
40. Kamei, M., Sato, H., Kamisawa, R., Yonemoto, K., Odashima, Y.: Audiol. Jpn. **63**(4), 272 (2020)
41. Ando, A., Imai, T., Kobayashi, A., Homma, S., Goto, J., Seiyama, N., Mishima, T., Kobayakawa, T., Sato, S., Onoe, K., et al.: IEICE Trans. Inf. Systems D-2. **86**(1), 15 (2003)
42. Homma, S., Kobayashi, A., Oku, T., Sato, S., Imai, T., Takagi, T.: J. Inst. Image Inf. Telev. Eng. **63**(3), 331 (2009)
43. Nakayama, T.: J. Inst. Electr. Eng. Jpn. **133**(9), 624 (2013)
44. Lasecki, W., Miller, C., Sadilek, A., Abumoussa, A., Borrello, D., Kushalnagar, R., Bigham, J.: Proceedings of the 25th Annual ACM Symposium on User Interface Software and Technology, pp. 23–34 (2012)
45. Miyoshi, S., Kawano, S., Shirasawa, M., Isoda, K., Ikarashi, Y.: J. Life Support Eng. **27**(3), 79 (2015)
46. UDTalk. https://udtalk.jp/en/
47. KoeTra app support page.. https://www.koetra.jp/en/
48. Matsuda, S., Hayashi, T., Ashikari, Y., Shiga, Y., Kashioka, H., Yasuda, K., Okuma, H., Uchiyama, M., Sumita, E., Kawai, H., et al.: IEICE Trans. Inf. Syst. **100**(4), 621 (2017)
49. Nakano, S., Makihara, T., Kanazawa, T., Nakano, Y., Arai, T., Kuroki, H., Ino, S., Ifukube, T.: IEICE Trans. Inf. Syst. **J90-D**(3), 808 (2007)
50. Sato, K., Takahashi, N., Hato, N.: Audiol. Jpn. **59**(1), 42 (2016)
51. Huenerfauth, M., Kacorri, H.: J. Technol. Pers. Disabil. **3**, 20 (2015)
52. Sharpe, R., Benfield, G., Roberts, G., Francis, R.: The Higher Education Academy. **4**(2), 24 (2006)
53. Hashim, H., Tasir, Z., Mohamad, S.K.: Turk. Online J. Educ. Technol. **12**(4), 67 (2013)
54. Farhan, W., Razmak, J.: Disabil. Rehabil. Assist. Technol. **17**(4), 431 (2022)
55. Bell, D., Foiret, J.: Disabil. Rehabil. Assist. Technol. **15**(7), 838 (2020)
56. Blatt, J., Rosch, G., Osterer, C.: IEEE Trans. Consum. Electron. (4), 717 (1980)
57. Othman, A., El Ghoul, O., Jemni, M.: Computers Helping People with Special Needs: 12th International Conference, ICCHP 2010, Vienna, Austria, July 14–16, 2010, Proceedings, Part II 12, pp. 169–176. Springer (2010)
58. Uchida, T., Sumiyoshi, H., Miyazaki, T., Azuma, M., Umeda, S., Kato, N., Hiruma, N., Kaneko, H., Yamanouchi, Y.: ITE Trans. Media Technol. Appl. **7**(3), 126 (2019)

59. Shibasaki, M., Kamiyama, Y., Minamizawa, K.: Adjunct Proceedings of the 29th Annual ACM Symposium on User Interface Software and Technology, pp. 97–99 (2016)
60. Peñeñory, V.M., Manresa-Yee, C., Riquelme, I., Collazos, C.A., Fardoun, H.M., Alghazzawi, D.M.: Proceedings of the 4th Workshop on ICTs for Improving Patients Rehabilitation Research Techniques, pp. 81–84 (2016)
61. Jiajun, Y., Zhiwu, Z., Meng, H., Yuexiang, L.: 2021 International Conference on Information Technology and Contemporary Sports (TCS), pp. 24–29. IEEE (2021)
62. Elvitigala, D.S., Wessolek, D., Achenbach, A.V., Singhabahu, C., Nanayakkara, S.: Proceedings of the 28th Australian Conference on Computer-Human Interaction, pp. 567–570 (2016)
63. Shitara, A., Namatame, M., Sarcar, S., Ochiai, Y., Shiraishi, Y.: Int. J. Hum.-Comput. Stud. **182**, 103168 (2024)

Chapter 10
Assisting Visually Impaired People: Sports and eSports

Takahiro Miura and Toshiaki Tanaka

Abstract Section 10.1: Parasports and accessible esports are advancing quickly as tools and frameworks expand participation among people with disabilities. Parasports originated from postwar rehabilitation at Stoke Mandeville and have grown into global, highly competitive events, including sports for athletes with visual impairments like goalball. Research shows physiological, psychological, and social benefits, which inform evidence-based training. In accessible esports, the growth of gaming platforms and audio-first design has increased opportunities for blind and low-vision players, supported by guidelines, codesign methods, screen readers, adaptive controllers, and accessible mainstream titles. Remaining gaps include localization, discoverability of features, refund policies, and nonvisual navigation challenges.

Section 10.2: This section highlights the growing application of eSports in rehabilitation for cognitive, motor, and social benefits, particularly among older adults and individuals with disabilities. In Japan and Western countries, eSports are used for upper limb training, attention enhancement, and balance improvement through virtual reality (VR). Institutions such as the Mayo Clinic support eSports medicine, while Japan integrates universal design devices in care facilities. Despite its benefits, risks such as overuse injuries, sensory overload, and game dependency require careful management. With proper support systems, eSports show promise for future rehabilitation, especially in post-pandemic and disaster recovery settings.

Section 10.3: This section surveys parasports for people with visual impairments and the assistive systems that support them. We outline adaptations of mainstream sports (e.g., guide running, tappers, tandem cycling, audible balls) and Paralympic participation, including vision classes (B1–B3) and athlete status categories. We

T. Miura
Research Institute on Human and Societal Augmentation (RIHSA), National Institute of Advanced Industrial Science and Technology (AIST), Chiba, Japan
e-mail: miura-t@aist.go.jp

T. Tanaka (✉)
Research Center for Advanced Science and Technology / Institute of Gerontology, The University of Tokyo, Tokyo, Japan
e-mail: t.tanaka@iog.u-tokyo.ac.jp; tanaka@bfp.rcast.u-tokyo.ac.jp

T. Tanaka (ed.), *Inclusive and Barrier-Free Designs for Rehabilitation Engineering*,
https://doi.org/10.1007/978-981-95-5783-7_10

identify three design themes—real-time assistance, performance optimization, and inclusive participation—and present *GoalBaural* as a case study: a binaural, VR-style trainer that enhanced directional and distance judgments. We then connect to accessible and para eSports, organizing current work into four strands—audio games, exergames, partially accessible mainstream titles, and inclusive co-play—along with tools, authoring environments, and community practices.

10.1 History and Development of Sports and eSports

10.1.1 Introduction, History, and Development of Parasports

To promote social participation among people with disabilities, progress has been made in developing and implementing tools and frameworks to support their activities. Especially in parasports and para eSports, rapid developments have occurred since the 2010s and 2020s, respectively. This chapter provides an overview of the current state of sports and eSports for individuals with disabilities.

Parasports (also known as disability sports or adaptive sports) originated as therapeutic gymnastics for individuals with sensory and physical impairments. The foundation of modern parasports can be traced to the establishment of the spinal injury unit at Stoke Mandeville Hospital (United Kingdom) in 1944, where Sir Ludwig Guttmann pioneered the innovative use of sports in rehabilitation [1–3]. He incorporated sports, especially archery, into treatment for spinal cord injury patients, showing significant benefits for neuromuscular health, increased patient motivation, and stronger camaraderie [4, 5]. This comprehensive approach involved early admission, prevention, and treatment of complications related to spinal cord injury, active rehabilitation, and social reintegration. The International Stoke Mandeville Games (ISMG) began in 1948 as a rehabilitation competition for injured veterans [6, 7]. The inaugural event featured 16 participants and was deliberately scheduled to coincide with the London Olympics. Initially characterized by strong recreational elements, the ISMG expanded significantly by 1952 when Dutch veterans joined British participants, with attendance growing to 130 competitors and establishing the first international competition of its kind [2].

The 1960 ISMG held in Rome is recognized as the first Paralympic Games [8, 9]. The term "Paralympic" was coined during the 1964 Tokyo Olympics, originally meaning "Paraplegia + Olympic," reflecting the initially focused on individuals with paraplegia. As participation expanded to include individuals with visual impairments and other disabilities beyond paraplegia, the meaning evolved to "Para (from Parallel) + Olympic," signifying games held parallel to the Olympics [10].

The formal integration of Olympic and Paralympic Games began with the 1988 Seoul Olympics, when the International Olympic Committee (IOC) officially recognized "Paralympic" as the formal designation for these competitions [6]. The development from the modest beginnings at Seoul 1988 with 18 sports, 732 events, and 3057 participants to the 2020 Tokyo Games (held in 2021) featuring 22 sports, 540 events, and 4403 participants, and the 2024 Paris Games with 22 sports and 549 events, demonstrates the remarkable growth and increasing competitiveness of Paralympic sports [11]. Parasports, which began as a therapeutic exercise for individuals with various sensory and physical disabilities and impairments, are becoming increasingly popular and competitive worldwide through international competitions, such as the Paralympic Games [12, 13].

During this evolutionary process, parasports transformed from therapeutic rehabilitation tools to recreational activities and ultimately to highly competitive athletic pursuits. Modern Paralympic Games include sports with visual impairment categories such as goalball, cycling (tandem), judo, blind football, rowing (blind sailing), triathlon, swiming, and athletics particularly in summer games. For example, goalball, specifically designed for athletes with visual impairments, was invented in 1946 as a form of rehabilitation for World War II veterans who lost their sight, and it made its Paralympic debut at the 1976 Games in Toronto [14]. Research on goalball has demonstrated the effectiveness of sports in developing unique perceptual abilities and coordination skills specific to athletes with visual impairments [15, 16].

Building upon this rich historical foundation and modern accessibility frameworks, parasports have evolved beyond mere medical intervention to serve crucial roles in promoting social participation, providing opportunities for self-realization, and advancing the creation of an inclusive society. Contemporary research continues to investigate the physiological, psychological, and social benefits of Paralympic sports, contributing to evidence-based approaches for optimizing training, performance, and athlete development in various disability categories [17–19].

10.1.2 History and Development of Accessible eSports (Para eSports)

The computer gaming market has experienced rapid growth worldwide and will continue expanding immediately in the coming years; the Global Games Market Report 2020 and 2024 estimated that the gaming population would reach 2.7 billion in 2020 and 3.4 billion in 2024 [20, 21]. In the year 2024, mobile games dominate the gaming demographic: the estimated player populations for console games, personal computer (PC) games, and mobile games are 630 million, 908 million, and 2848 million, respectively [21]. The population of computer game players currently spans a wider range of age groups. This trend might be due to the global coronavirus disease 2019 (COVID-19) pandemic, which led to government *stay-at-home* orders and social distancing measures in many countries [22], causing demand for computer games to soar.

Since the advent of computer games in the 1970s, the history of gaming has already exceeded half a century. Initially, games were available in commercial venues like amusement arcades that housed arcade cabinets. However, in the 1980s, the development and sale of home video game consoles using software cartridges, such as the *ATARI 2600* (or *ATARI* Video Computer System (VCS)), *Nintendo Entertainment System* (NES) (or Nintendo *Family Computer* in Japan), and Sega *Genesis* (or *Mega Drive* in Japan), drove rapid growth. During the 1990s and 2000s, handheld game consoles like the Nintendo *Game Boy* and Sega *Game Gear* emerged, followed by the widespread availability of games on mobile devices. Additionally, platforms for playing *exergames* (exercise + games), such as the Nintendo *Wii*, had emerged, expanding the player base. From the 2000s to the 2010s, touchscreen mobile devices such as smartphones and tablets (Apple *iPhone/iPad*, Google *Pixel*, etc.) became common, allowing users to play games on these devices. Today, in the 2020s, not only young people but also older adults are playing games daily more than ever.

From the perspective of enjoyable games especially for visually impaired people, there were almost no games available for them to play in the 1980s. In the 1990s, Warp Co., Ltd. introduced the *Real Sound* genre, which could be played using only sound, and even provided braille instruction manuals to those who requested them, making it possible for visually impaired people to play the mainstream games. They released a game called "Real Sound: Kaze no Regret" (roughly translated as "Real Sound: The Wind's Regret") for the Sega Saturn in 1997. However, the game did not achieve commercial success, and no other games in the Real Sound genre have been released since.

However, due to the growth of game content and the technological advances in hardware performance and software capabilities, the number of games accessible to people with visual impairments increased in the late 1990s and early 2000s, irrespective of whether the game platform is stationary or portable. On the websites *AudioGames.net* and *accessible game wiki* (in Japanese), volunteers who are enthusiastic gamers with visual impairments share information on playable and non-playable games independently or with assistance [23, 24]. Besides the information on audio games mentioned earlier, these websites also share details about games that are playable due to their rich sound effects. In the author's immediate circle, there are several blind individuals who play *Pokémon* (Nintendo, Game Freak, and Creatures). In Pokémon, each of the hundreds of fictional creatures has a unique sound effect (or cry), allowing players to identify their species based on the cries. When learning to associate sounds with in-game events, some visually impaired players reportedly receive assistance from sighted individuals. In this context, they also participate in cooperative play and competitive matches.

Entering the 2020s, the accumulation of knowledge from various game accessibility guidelines proposed particularly in the 2010s [25–29], the establishment of various legal systems, and the expansion of player demographics as well as the proposals of game codesigning methods involving persons with disabilities [30] have led to the emergence of many mainstream games enjoyably playable regardless of age or disability. At the game console level, screen reader functionality has been implemented in the *PlayStation 5* (released in November 2020) and *Nintendo Switch 2* (released in June 2025), and accessibility improvements are progressing on PC game platforms such as *Steam*. Moreover, controllers for people with physical disabilities have appeared, such as the *Xbox Adaptive Controller* (Microsoft), *PS5 Access Controller* (Sony), and *Flex Controller* (HORI). Titles with improved accessibility for visually impaired players include Naughty Dog's *The Last of Us Part I* (remake version released in September 2022) and *The Last of Us Part II* (June 2020, with a remastered version released in November 2023 featuring accessible audio guides), *Marvel's Spider-Man 2* whose developer is the Insomniac Games (October 2023), and *Diablo IV* by the Blizzard Entertainment (June 2024). Additionally, titles like *Street Fighter 6* by the Capcom (June 2023), which includes sound accessibility features (such as conveying the distance and health status of opponents through sound effects), and the digital card game *Hearthstone* by the Blizzard Entertainment (March 2014), which supports screen readers, allow visually impaired players to compete against sighted players in eSports. However, as of 2025, some issues with insufficient accessibility localization were identified, such as the text-to-speech functionality being available only in English and not in Japanese. Even when options like larger subtitles or color adjustments are provided, users may still find it challenging to navigate the game space using senses other than vision, leading to difficulties in progressing the game. The availability of accessibility features can also be difficult to identify before purchasing, and some stores do not offer refunds, leaving users who need accessibility features without a trustworthy way to buy games confidently.

Summary

Section 10.1: Parasports and accessible esports are advancing quickly as tools and frameworks expand participation among people with disabilities. Parasports originated from postwar rehabilitation at Stoke Mandeville and have grown into global, highly competitive events, including sports for athletes with visual impairments like goalball. Research shows physiological, psychological, and social benefits, which inform evidence-based training. In accessible esports, the growth of gaming platforms and audio-first design has increased opportunities for blind and low-vision players, supported by guidelines, codesign methods, screen readers, adaptive controllers, and accessible mainstream titles. Remaining gaps include localization, discoverability of features, refund policies, and nonvisual navigation challenges.

10.2 Application of eSports in Rehabilitation

10.2.1 Background

eSports (electronic sports) have expanded globally since the spread of PC and console games in the 1990s. In recent years, they have been introduced in elderly care facilities and medical institutions, showing diverse applications that go beyond mere entertainment [31]. Particularly in Western countries, eSports have been applied in rehabilitation for purposes such as cognitive training, improvement of reaction speed, and upper limb motor training [32].

In Japan, the adoption of eSports in elderly welfare facilities is accelerating as part of recreational and health promotion initiatives (Japan eSports Care Association, 2021 [33]). Japan initially lagged in the industrialization of eSports, with legal constraints (such as gambling regulations on prize competitions) hindering growth until the late 2010s. However, according to a survey by Japan eSports Union (JeSU), the domestic eSports market grew from approximately 4.8 billion yen in 2018 to over 10 billion yen in 2022, with tournaments such as *Shadowverse* and *PUBG MOBILE* awarding over 1 billion yen in total prizes [34] (Greenberg Traurig).

Meanwhile, in the fields of rehabilitation and welfare, cases in which elderly and disabled individuals maintain and recover physical and cognitive functions through gaming have attracted attention. Universal design-based eSports equipment developed by the UDe-Sports Association has been introduced into approximately 120 care and welfare facilities [35] (smartlaunch.com).

In the West, particularly in the United States, the Department of Physical Medicine and Rehabilitation (PM&R) began focusing on eSports medicine in the early 2020s. At the Mayo Clinic, the Gaming and Esports Medicine (GEM) team provides comprehensive services including posture correction, prevention and treatment of overuse injuries (e.g., tendinitis, tendon sheath inflammation in the elbow and wrist, lower back pain), lifestyle guidance, as well as nutritional and psychological support [36].

10.2.2 History and Current Status of Sports Medicine in eSports

Since the late 1990s, eSports have developed into formal competitive events, and by the 2000s, international tournaments became widespread. However, in the early stages, physical strain and health effects on players were largely overlooked. From the 2010s onward, concerns have grown over prolonged sitting posture, eye strain, and repetitive stress injuries (especially carpal tunnel syndrome and tendinitis), as well as psychological issues such as insomnia and burnout. These factors prompted researchers to begin studying eSports within the framework of sports medicine (DiFrancisco- Donoghue et al. 2019 [37]).

Today, the importance of conditioning, physical exercise interventions, neurophysiological effects of visual and auditory stimuli, and mental health support for eSports players is widely recognized. In particular, in Western countries, progress has been made in providing rehabilitation and preventive medical support. For example, the American College of Sports Medicine (ACSM) has proposed that eSports athletes require "exercise prescriptions" such as stretching, strength training, and posture correction [38]. Furthermore, collaboration between physical therapists and sports psychologists has been advancing to support both performance enhancement and long-term health maintenance [39].

10.2.3 Application to Rehabilitation

When applying eSports to rehabilitation, a multifaceted approach is important, one that targets physical function recovery, cognitive maintenance and enhancement, and psychosocial activation. The following are some examples of its applications.

- Upper Limb Motor Training: Games using controllers, mice, or touch screens require repetitive hand and arm movements. For example, tablet-based game applications allow hemiplegic patients to repeat reaching motions and screen tapping, potentially expanding their range of motion through repetition and improving concentration.
- Attention and Reaction Training: Fighting and music games demand instantaneous judgment and reaction to visual and auditory stimuli, thus contributing to improved attention and processing speed (Bavelier et al. 2008) [40]. In particular, rhythm games that require physical movement in tempo can serve as integrated cognitive-motor training, with potential use in rehabilitation for cognitive impairments poststroke and attention decline in older adults [41].
- Promotion of Social Interaction: In care facilities and day services, implementing competitive or team-based games among older adults can stimulate motivation and a sense of competition, which in turn may lead to greater engagement in daily life (Japan eSports Care Association 2021) [33].
- Balance and Lower Limb Training (VR based): Games that integrate VR devices (e.g., Oculus Quest 2 and PlayStation VR) with balance boards or accelerometer sensors can help train lower limb strength and postural control. Games that require body and leg movements (e.g., Beat Saber) simultaneously stimulate multiple sensory systems, which may contribute to improvements in dynamic balance (Bieleke 2025) [42]. Furthermore, the immersive nature of the gaming environment may enhance motivation to participate in rehabilitation.

The VR games currently being worked on in Tanaka Laboratory are for children with severe physical and mental disabilities. Three are trunk and upper limb training game that can be played from a wheelchair (Figs. 10.1, 10.2, and 10.3). As these children are severely disabled, rehabilitation using games that can be played from a wheelchair or bed is an important rehabilitation method for maintaining and improving their motivation of disabled children and preventing a decline in limb and trunk function. Table 10.1 summarizes examples of the use of eSports in rehabilitation.

According to the risk management for eSports-based rehabilitation, it is important to manage physical and cognitive risks, as well as potential dependency. Key risks and countermeasures include the following.

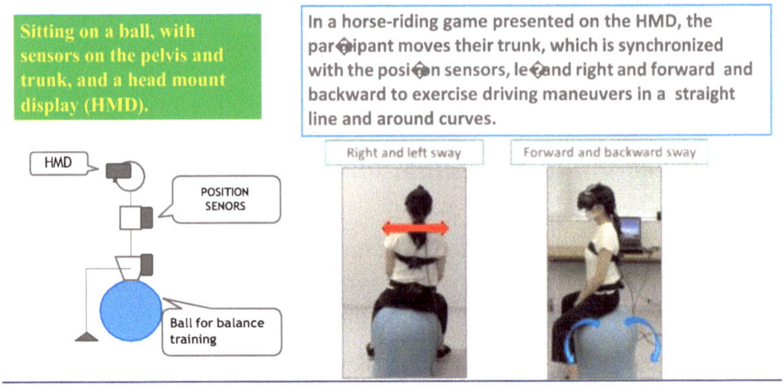

Fig. 10.1 VR rehabilitation for the trunk training using a HMD system

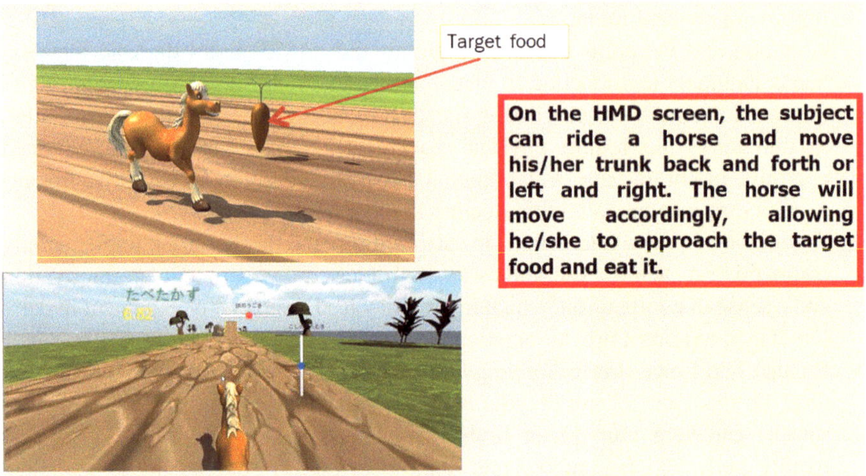

Fig. 10.2 VR rehabilitation game for the trunk training while riding a horse

- Risk of Overuse and Muscle Fatigue: Even for therapeutic purposes, extended continuous gameplay may lead to muscle fatigue, joint overload, and decreased concentration. Particularly for patients with limited upper limb function, conditions such as tendinitis of the elbow or shoulder may arise. Sessions should be limited to 20–30 min with breaks and ideally supervised by therapists who evaluate joint pain and fatigue levels afterward.
- Visual and Auditory Overload: eSports involve intense visual and auditory stimulation, which may cause eye strain or hypersensitivity to sounds over long periods. Adjust screen brightness appropriately and prefer external speakers to earphones to reduce the acoustic pressure risk.
- Fall Risk (in VR environments): Standing games in VR can increase the risk of falls owing to spatial misperception or loss of balance. Play areas should be

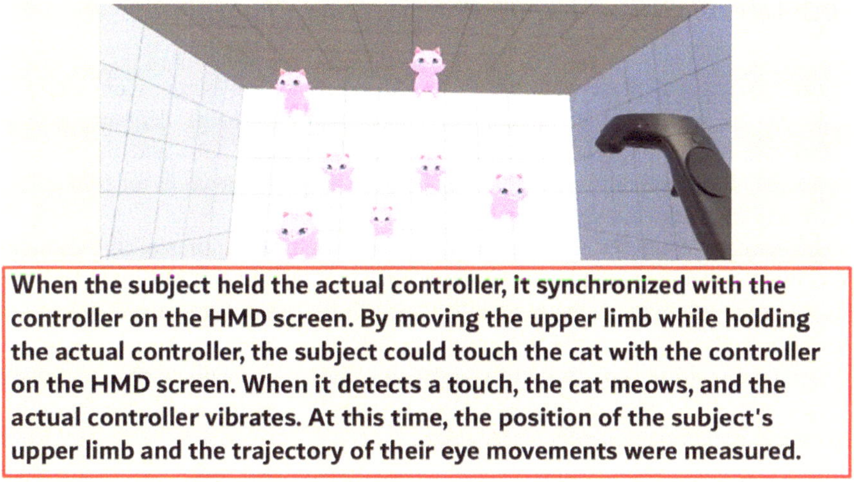

Fig. 10.3 VR rehabilitation game for upper limbs

Table 10.1 Examples of eSports applications in rehabilitation (mapped by body area/function)

Target function	Applicable eSports	Effect
Upper limb range of motion and dexterity	Racing games, shooting games	Shoulder, elbow, wrist, finger movements
Reaction speed and attention	Fighting games, music games	Cognitive and reaction training
Balance sense and lower limb strength	VR sports, Wii Fit	Balance training and gait assistance
Social interaction and motivation	Online team-based games	QOL improvement through communication and interaction

cleared of obstacles, and mats or cushions should be placed on the floor. Therefore, the presence of caregivers was recommended. For those with difficulty in standing, game titles were chosen from a seated position.

- Risk of Dependency or Overfocus on Gaming: For users with cognitive decline or developmental disorders, there is a risk of becoming overly engrossed in games and deviating from the original rehabilitation goals. It is essential to define time and frequency clearly as structured training tasks and establish a monitoring system with therapists or family members.
- Difficulty Operating Devices and Learning Burden: Game operation may be psychologically challenging for the elderly or cognitively impaired users. Use color-coded controller buttons, provide large-font visual guides, and simplify the user interface (UI). Pre-experience sessions or trial periods before formal introduction can help reduce anxiety and improve confidence in participation.

10.2.4 Conclusion: Future Prospects and Challenges

While eSports can place both physical and psychological burdens on users, its strategic use as a form of rehabilitation is increasingly being demonstrated. In Japan, the use of eSports in welfare contexts for older adults and people with disabilities is progressing, but medical and rehabilitation frameworks for competitive players remain under development.

In Western countries, eSports players are treated as legitimate athletes, with rehabilitation and preventive care systems already institutionalized. Going forward, it will be important for Japan to establish specialized "eSports medicine" teams and strengthen education and research infrastructure in this area.

Furthermore, the application of eSports in elderly care facilities and support for people with disabilities in the post-COVID era, as well as its use in disaster or war recovery support, is also gaining attention.

10.3 Parasports and Its Support Systems

10.3.1 Parasports for Visually Impaired People

Adapted physical activity refers to existing mainstream sports that people with disabilities cannot participate in, modified by adjusting rules, equipment, and methods to meet the needs of the participants. This concept is also applied to parasports for people with visual impairments (Table 10.2).

In parasports, the Paralympic Games include 28 sports—22 summer and 6 winter. Competitors with visual impairments can participate in the following 12 sports—9 summer and 3 winter.

Summer Track and field, cycling, equestrian, goalball, judo, paratriathlon, rowing, soccer (five-a-side, a.k.a., blind soccer), and swimming

Winter Alpine skiing and Nordic skiing, such as biathlon and cross country

Additionally, while not included in the Paralympic Games, sports commonly played by visually impaired individuals include ball games such as volleyball (e.g., *floor volleyball*), softball (e.g., *grand softball*), and tennis (e.g., *blind tennis*), as well as individual sports like *paraclimbing*. In table tennis, there are several variations, such as *swish* (developed by an Australian person with blindness), *showdown* (developed by a Canadian person with blindness), and *sound table tennis* (STT) (devised by a Japanese educator). These variations commonly use audible balls, such as a ball with a bell (*swish* and SST) or BBs (*showdown*) inside, and involve hitting the ball under the net instead of over it, but differ in the shape of the table and rackets and game rules. Note that when using the term "para table tennis," the main players are athletes with physical disabilities and intellectual impairments, not those with

Table 10.2 Examples of adaptations on mainstream sports for visually impaired players [43]

Sport	Examples of accommodations
Track and field	Side-by-side running with guide runners holding a guide rope and providing audio cues
Swimming	Tapping by an experienced guide tapper who signals turns and finishes
Judo	Beginning the competition after grappling
Cycling	Using tandem bicycles, with the sighted pilot controlling from the front seat
Skiing	Providing a guide that offers information while moving in front of or beside the athlete to replace visual cues
Ball game	*Rules*: Often use space as a flat surface and maintain silence during competition *Equipment*: Auditory information from the ball, three-dimensional lines, contrasting colors *Safety*: Fences along the sidelines *Information*: Providing information support through sighted callers, etc.

Table 10.3 Visual impairment classification on Paralympic sports [45]

Levels	Visual acuity	Visual field
B1	logMAR: >2.6 (decimal: <0.0025, Snellen: <20/7962)	None
B2	logMAR: 1.5–2.6 (decimal: 0.0025–0.032, Snellen: 20/632–20/7962)	Diameter < 10°
B3	logMAR: 1.0–1.4 (decimal: 0.04–0.1, Snellen: 20/200–20/502)	Diameter < 40°

visual impairments, and the equipment and game rules are nearly the same as in regular table tennis.

In parasports, athletes are classified based on their disability conditions according to the International Paralympic Committee (IPC) Classification Code [44, 45]. The visually impaired are divided into three categories—B1, B2, and B3 in order of severity—according to visual acuity and visual field (Table 10.3). For visual acuity, athletes with corrected decimal visual acuity of 0.1 (which equals Snellen visual acuity of 20/200 or logMAR visual acuity of 1.0) or less in the better eye are eligible to participate in competitions. Visual field is assessed using the Goldman perimetry III/4e index. Additionally, athletes are evaluated on their status, which indicates how long they are eligible to compete in a specific category [44]. They are classified into four statuses: confirmed (C), review at the next available opportunity (R-NAO), review with a fixed review date (R-FRD), and expired (E). C does not require additional evaluation except in cases of regulation changes. R-NAO mandates the completion of an evaluation session prior to participating in any competition. R-FRD permits participation in competitions until the predetermined review date; however, it necessitates the completion of an evaluation session before participating in subsequent competitions. E is not eligible to participate in competitions unless they undergo an evaluation again.

10.3.2 Assistive Systems and Support Applications for Parasports and Physical Activity

Across visually impaired parasports, assistive systems and support applications focus on three main themes:

1. *Real-time assistance*: audio-haptic guidance for navigation, positioning, pacing, lane keeping and wall approach, and collision avoidance during training and competition
2. *Performance optimization*: technique analysis, training feedback, and skill development through biomechanical assessment, sensor-based workload monitoring, and injury risk management
3. *Inclusive participation*: systems that enhance social interaction, spectator experience, and community engagement in parasports (e.g., public tryout/education settings)

Representative examples include sonified navigation and cue-design guidelines [46], wearable workload monitoring [47], maintaining body balance and mobility [48, 49], running guidance and line-following support [50–52], swimming aids using audio or vibrotactile cues [53, 54], goalball analytics and impact/load quantification [55–57], and outreach-oriented systems and workshops that broaden participation [58–60].

10.3.3 Goalball and Training Application of the Aural Sense

This section describes an example of performance optimization, specifically an auditory training support system for goalball developed by the author and colleagues, along with its effects.

10.3.3.1 Overview

Goalball is a team sport comprising three players on each side, specifically designed for athletes with visual impairments. The game is conducted on an indoor court that measures identically to a standard volleyball court. Two teams, each consisting of three players equipped with eyeshades, employ a specialized ball weighing 1.25 kg, which contains bells inside. The objective of the game is to throw the ball across the opposing team's goal line as frequently as possible, while defenders from the opposing team endeavor to intercept the ball using their bodies.

Recent research on goalball has increasingly emphasized its health promotion benefits and performance improvement strategies. A scoping review by Petrigna et al. showed that goalball athletes experience decreases in body fat and body mass index (BMI), as well as improvements in cardiorespiratory endurance, muscular strength, muscular endurance, and flexibility [61]. Additionally, positive effects on postural control and auditory reaction speed were observed compared to sedentary individuals with visual impairments. Particularly, Karakaya et al. found that goalball players significantly outperformed their non-active peers in body composition (body mass index, skinfold thickness of triceps plus calf), musculoskeletal function (trunk lift, curl up, and isometric push-up), aerobic function (1-mile run/walk test), and anaerobic power (vertical jump) [62]. Effective balance improvement in goalball players has also been reported in another systematic review by Palacín Artigosa et al. [63]. Makaracı et al. identified significant correlations between postural stability, physical fitness level, and shooting accuracy in Paralympic-level female goalball players, suggesting a connection between balance training and competitive performance [64].

Performance enhancement has been studied concerning the relationship between physiological parameters and technical performance. Alves et al. examined the links between aerobic and anaerobic parameters and game technical performance in elite goalball athletes [65]. Regarding biomechanical insights for skill development, Gökşen et al. analyzed muscle activation patterns during goalball throwing movements, showing ball velocity is primarily related to upper extremity flexor muscle strength rather than visual acuity [66]. Larsen's reported psychological interventions included a six-step mental skill training program—preliminary meeting, initiation, maintenance of the process and motivation, arousal and prep for competition, creating a winning mentality, and championship prep—applied to Denmark's women's team, demonstrating strategies' effectiveness in disability sports [67]. These findings collectively demonstrate that goalball enhances physical abilities and social participation for individuals with visual impairments, supporting evidence-based training.

10.3.3.2 GoalBaural: Application for Training Aural Sense for Goalball Players

Since goalball players cannot rely on visual information, they must perceive the game dynamics through auditory cues. Nonetheless, perceiving the positions of opponents, as well as the direction and distance of the incoming ball, can be particularly challenging, especially for novice players. Furthermore, inexperienced players often experience fear of high-speed approaching balls due to the risk of injury associated with the absence of visual guidance. Additionally, there is a limited availability of environments suitable for practicing defensive techniques. Thus, the author introduces an example of our developed acoustic virtual reality (VR) system named *GoalBaural* (a name combining "goalball" and "aural"), which enables users to independently perform comprehensive goalball training without visiting the gym [68, 69].

GoalBaural [68] (and GoalBaural-II [69]) enables users to train their sound localization ability for scenarios such as a ball being thrown from various directions to different locations. GoalBaural first presents the binaural sound of the throw and then asks the user to identify the exact direction and distance for defense. This application was developed by recording the throwing sound binaurally with a dummy head microphone and then designing an interface to play sounds randomly and evaluate the user's reactions. The dummy head was used for recording because accurately capturing moving sounds is challenging with traditional methods like convolution of moving sounds with head-related transfer functions (HRTFs) or head-related impulse responses (HRIRs) [70].

10.3.4 Binaural Recording of Sounds

The environmental setup for the sound recording is illustrated in Fig. 10.4. The dummy head microphone (Southern Acoustics, SAMREC Type 2500s conforming to the standards IEC 60959 and IEC 60268-7) was used to record sound in various situations, including throws.

In the case of throws, the time-series sounds included the approach run for throwing the ball, the throw, and the ball passing horizontally. The dummy head was positioned at the center of the line, 3 m from the edge, with the height of its external ear canals at 65 cm from the floor, placed inside a goalball coat in a

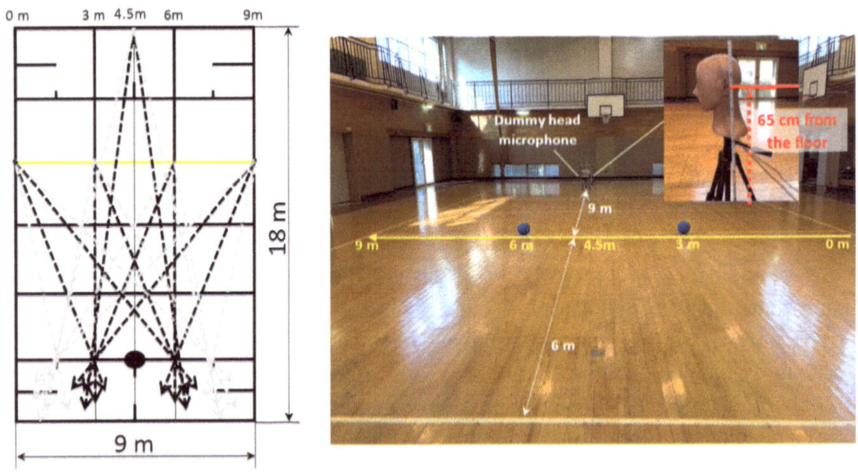

Fig. 10.4 Recording setup of throwing sound of the ball of goalball. (Left) This is a schematic bird's-eye view of the recording setup. The black circle indicates the dummy head microphone, and dash lines represent the trajectory of the player's runway and throw of the ball. (Right) Photograph of the recording setup. The yellow line corresponds to the yellow line in the left figure

university gym (background noise level (L_{Aeq}): 45.6 dBA; reverberation time: 1.8 s). The 65-cm height reflects the typical head height of a player during play. This dummy head was used to record the sound of a moving competition ball (KSG Goalball) thrown by three partially blind players who have participated in this sport for over a year and play regularly.

One of the participants was asked to start running straight from a distance of 15 m in front of the dummy head and then throw the ball at the 9-m line (yellow line illustrated in the left part of Fig. 10.4) from the dummy head. At that time, the participant threw the ball at 0, 3, 4.5, 6, and 9 m from the right edge line shown in the right figure of Fig. 10.4 to make the ball skitter across the left or right side of the dummy head. The types of throws included grounders, meaning the ball rolls along the floor and bounces on the floor. The trajectories of the participants and the ball are illustrated as dashed lines in the left part of Fig. 10.4. When the thrower started to run on the left or right sides of the center vertical line, shown in the left figure of Fig. 10.4, the position of the dummy head microphone was displaced approximately 75 cm (near) or 150 cm (far) to the left or right of the center. In this case, the thrower was at 4.5 m from the right edge line, and the dummy head was also at the central location of the horizontal line, as shown in the left figure of Fig. 10.4. These place conditions of the dummy head simulated the practical positions of goalball experts in their competition games.

The recording was made using Audacity. The sound captured by the dummy head microphone was recorded through the audio interface (Roland Edirol UA-4FX) at a sampling rate of 48 kHz and a bit depth of 16 bits. After recording, it was determined that the time interval started from the participant's run until just before the ball hit the wall, based on the recorded sounds.

10.3.5 Application Implementation

GoalBaural is designed to assist individuals with visual impairments by providing randomized scenarios to help them learn to identify the positions of players, as well as the direction and distance of the ball during training. The system can operate within a Windows environment, with or without screen readers such as NVDA, Jaws, and PC Talker. Users listen through headphones to binaural sounds, and their responses can be recorded to determine correctness.

The upper and lower panels of Fig. 10.5 illustrate the GoalBaural user experience and display the interfaces for each state. When the user presses enter or space, a recorded binaural sound plays through the headphones after a brief silence of 1–6 s (version 1) or 1–2 s (version 2). This silent time simulates the experience of defenders in a real game, as they wait for sudden pitches. The user then must decide which side the virtual ball would pass from their first-person perspective. In GoalBaural version I, users press the F or J key to indicate the left or right side as quickly as possible. In version II, users determine the ball's travel direction and press

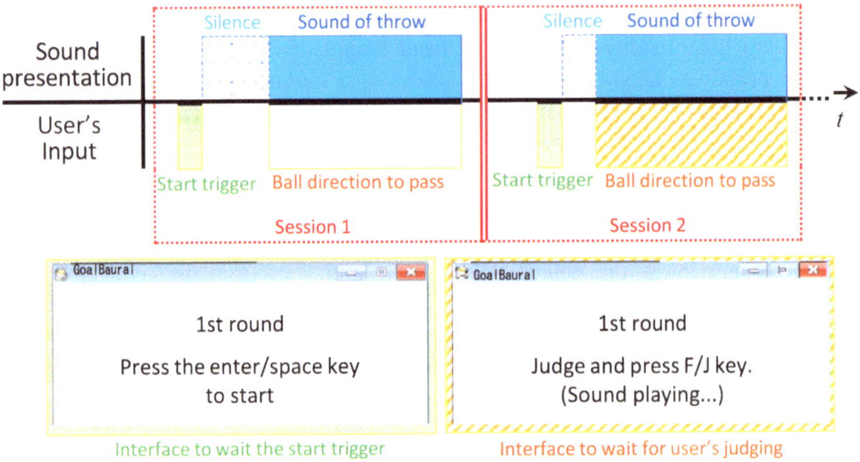

Fig. 10.5 (Upper) User experience procedure and (lower) interface of GoalBaural (version 1)

D/F or J/K for the left or right side. They press D and K when the ball's expected position is farther from the user on the defensive line compared to pressing F and J. If no key is pressed by the end of the sound, the next session begins after a short rest period, equal to half the sound duration.

10.3.6 Key Training Effects by GoalBaural

GoalBaural-II was evaluated by five participants with over 2 years of experience with goalball, including two with low vision and three who were blind, in their early 20s [69].

Figure 10.6a shows the correct response rates for ball direction increased with repetitions ($r = 0.46$, $p = 0.019$). Mean correct rates improved from 93.6% (first trial) to 100% (last trial). Despite the small participant group, significant main effects were observed for pitch trajectories and repetitions ($p = 0.018$ and $p = 0.004$, respectively), with straight throws achieving higher accuracy (98.7%) than crossing throws (95.6%). A significant three-way interaction among pitch distances, trajectories, and repetitions was also found ($p = 0.006$). Figure 10.6b displays correct response rates for ball direction and distance, showing improvement with repetitions ($r = 0.62$, $p < 0.001$). Mean accuracy increased from 55.2% to 86.4% between the first and last trials. Significant main effects were observed for pitch distances and repetitions, with multiple interactions detected ($p = 0.004$ to $p < 0.001$). Notably, accuracy improvement was greater for near pitches (36% increase) compared to far pitches (12% increase). Therefore, repetitions significantly enhanced accuracy in judging ball direction and distance, with training effects varying by pitch conditions and being more pronounced for near-distance pitches.

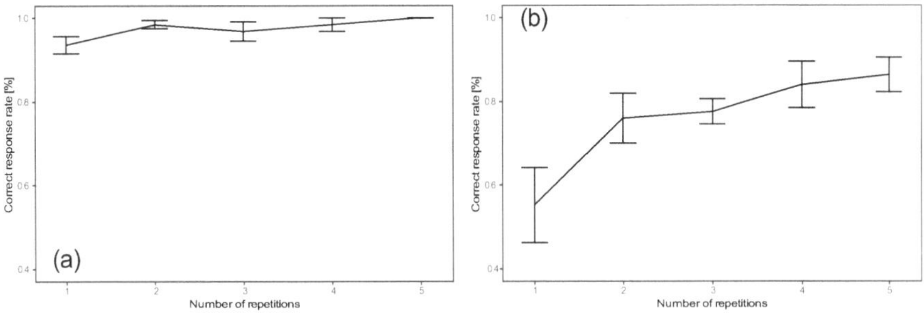

Fig. 10.6 Correct response rates regarding ball direction (**a**) and correct response rates regarding ball direction and distance (**b**) as a function of the number of repetitions

10.4 Para eSports and Accessible and Inclusive Games: Design, Evaluation, and Participation

Building on prior syntheses (e.g., [71–73]) that position disability, sport, and technology within broader participation agendas, research on para eSports and accessible games spans four overlapping strands: audio games, exergames, partially accessible mainstream titles, and inclusive games co-playable across sighted and blind and low-vision (BLV) players. Across these strands, assistive systems and support applications increasingly combine nonvisual feedback, input adaptations, and evaluation frameworks to improve both moment-to-moment play and longer-term skill development.

10.4.1 Audio Games

Research on audio games for BLV players has progressed through three waves. Early pioneers (pre-2010) demonstrated the feasibility of audio-first mechanics and genre preservation without visuals, such as rhythm-action adaptations using spatial sound and haptics [74] and instruction-free audio games showing learnability through interaction alone [75]. The transitional period (2010–2019) shifted toward controlled studies and transfer: the Audio-based Environment Simulator (AbES) line demonstrated that exploring a mapped building through audio games can enhance wayfinding and that learned layouts transfer to the physical environment, with methods and protocols documented for replication [76–80]. Meanwhile, design guidelines and empirical research have solidified best practices in audio-first level design and its affordances [81, 82]. Recent advances (2020–) establish audio games as a unique, adaptable design space: codesign studies with BLV players refine experience goals and mechanics [83], and novel rhythm-action systems demonstrate how feedback granularity can be adjusted without compromising challenge [84].

10.4.2 Exergames and Effort to Play Mainstream Games

Since around 2010, gaming devices such as the Nintendo *Wii Remote* (a.k.a. *Wiimote*) and Microsoft *Kinect*, which capture body movements, have become widely available, leading to an increase in research on *exergames* that visually impaired individuals can play using their bodies. Foundational examples include *VI-Tennis* and *VI-Bowling*, which utilize the Wiimote and vibrotactile timing cues, as well as earcons, to scaffold swinging and release actions [85, 86]. Complementary efforts targeted specific motor outcomes and pediatric contexts: *Pet-N-Punch* was an upper-body tactile/audio exergame that prompted vigorous arm actions and sustained participation from children who are blind [87]. Later work explored balance exergaming for blind children, using sensory substitution cues for postural control and showing promising feasibility for school-aged training [88]. Morelli and Folmer also proposed a sensory substitution process that detects key visual events like hurdles in Kinect exergames and converts them into vibrotactile cues, maintaining challenge while improving playability [89].

Instead of developing specialized games, researchers modify input/output pipelines so BLV players can access commercial titles. Examples include an affordable, accessible controller for 3D navigation [90] and audio-centric experiments in a mainstream open-world game [91]. Analytical tools help evaluate accessibility features on a large scale—both for individual titles (e.g., *The Last of Us Part II*) [92] and through two-step analysis workflows such as checklist review and user review analysis [93]. These tools complement broader arguments for the value of accessible games [71].

In some commercial games with inaccessible elements, visual information is replaced with auditory cues, often causing overload. Matsuo et al. developed a tactile game controller (*TactCon*) to reassign auditory and tactile information (see Figs. 10.7 and 10.8) and reported that using this controller significantly improves game completion [94]. To assess such gameplay, Miura et al. proposed a method based on difficulty adjustment using item response theory [95].

10.4.3 Inclusive Play and Development of Games and Gamers Community

Inclusive games and community initiatives span from co-playable board and digital games—where audio-haptic enhancements support mixed-ability groups [96]—to creator-facing tools that enable BLV authorship. In this context, Matsuo et al. created *AudibleMapper*, an authoring environment that lets blind creators build a map (Fig. 10.9) and developed an action role-playing game (RPG) *ShadowRine* playable through auditory and tactile feedback (Fig. 10.10) [97]. Beyond bespoke authoring, the ecosystem now includes accessible development workflows: coding

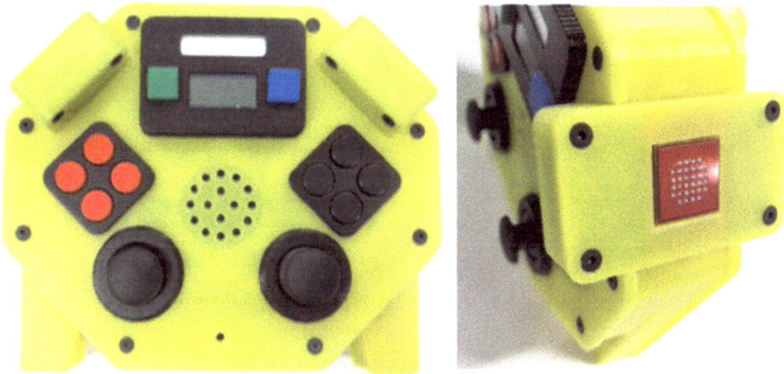

Fig. 10.7 Tactile game controller (*TactCon*) [94]

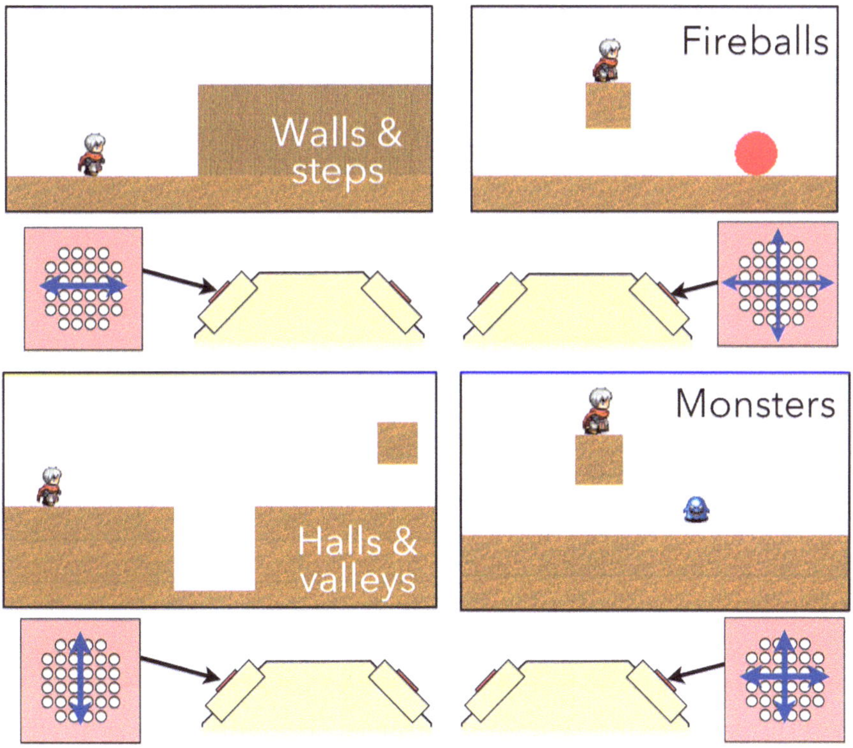

Fig. 10.8 Examples of the situations in the game and the corresponding tactile patterns presented by *TactCon* [94]

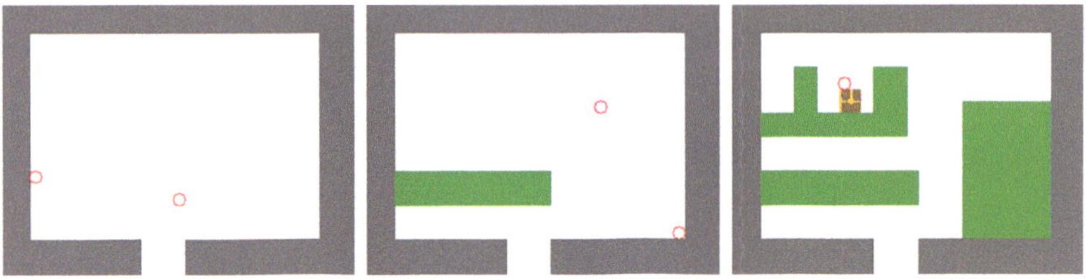

Fig. 10.9 An example of drawing with the *AudibleMapper* [97]. This tool displays the cursor's horizontal and vertical coordinates on the screen using interaural level differences and volume through headphones, respectively, and two-dimensional fields are created with keyboard operations. First, it begins with a map enclosed by walls on all four sides (left figure). Next, the walls are arranged to match the layout of the map (central figure). Lastly, objects like treasures are added (right figure). The red circles in the figure represent the cursor for editing

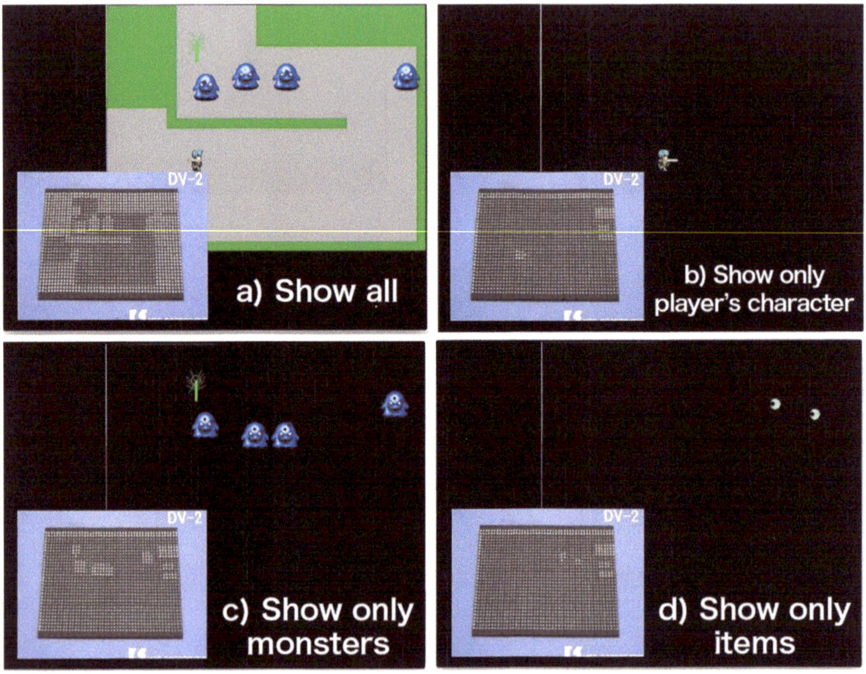

Fig. 10.10 Game views of *ShadowRine* and corresponding tactile outputs on a dot matrix display [98]

plug-ins that expose structure and intent to screen readers [99, 100], a grid-based coding paradigm designed for BLV programmers [101], accessible terminals optimized for screen reader interaction [102], and game engines/platforms supporting blind designers [103].

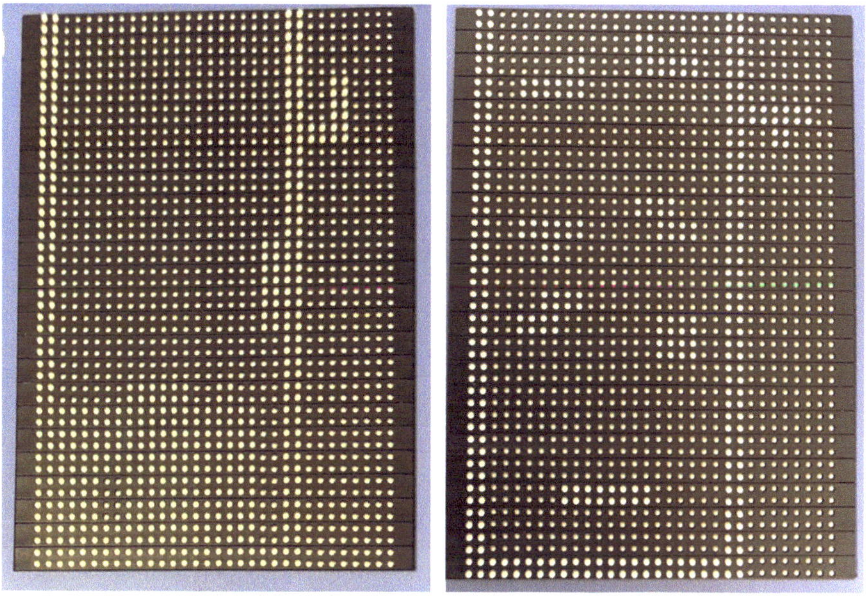

Fig. 10.11 (Left) Tactris play screen shown on a dot matrix display and (right) seven different types of tetrominoes [108]

On the community side, adoption studies surface persistent barriers (e.g., input complexity, social frictions) alongside motivations and difficulty-joy trade-offs [26, 104]. Inclusion has also expanded to spectatorship: game-aware streaming prototypes tailor broadcasts for BLV audiences [105]. Complementing these perspectives, usage research on BLV mobile gaming documents concrete strategies for overcoming inaccessible interfaces in the wild [106]. Finally, overarching frameworks synthesize design spaces and principles to make accessibility customizable and systematically integrated into play [107].

As of 2025, gaming environments where both sighted and visually impaired individuals can play and compete together will gradually be developed. *Tactris*, developed by the author's group, is a falling block puzzle game accessible to both users who cannot utilize tactile cues through a dot matrix display and those who depend on visual cues on the screen (Fig. 10.11) [108]. Seven types of tetrominoes (shapes composed of four squares) fall from the top of the screen, and players move and rotate them to fill gaps and score points. Blind players can increase their scores by using tactile feedback, and those with prior experience playing similar falling block puzzles before losing their sight are likely to benefit from tactile cues. Additionally, *Street Fighter 6* (Capcom) features sound accessibility options, allowing sighted players to enjoy the game without relying on visual cues [109]. This opens up opportunities for diverse and inclusive gameplay for individuals with and without disabilities.

10.4.4 Conclusion

This section discusses parasports designed for visually impaired athletes as adapted versions of common sports. Modifications include guide ropes on tracks, tappers in swimming, tandem cycling, and audible balls with silence rules in court games. Within the Paralympic system, athletes compete in vision classes B1–B3, with eligibility categorized as confirmed, review, or expired. Assistive technologies and support applications serve three main purposes: (1) providing real-time audio and haptic cues for navigation, pacing, lane maintenance, wall detection, and collision avoidance; (2) enhancing performance through biomechanical analysis, sensor-based workload tracking, and injury prevention; and (3) promoting inclusive participation via outreach, spectatorship, and co-playing. As a demonstration tool, GoalBaural utilizes binaural recordings of authentic goalball throws and randomized scenarios on Windows, compatible with screen readers. Tests showed improvements in directional accuracy (e.g., toward the ceiling) and combined direction-distance judgments, with larger gains observed for near throws.

Finally, these principles connect to para eSports. Current research and practice cover four areas—audio games, exergames, partially accessible mainstream titles, and inclusive co-play—supported by platform features and tools. Console-level screen readers (e.g., PS5, Switch 2), adaptive controllers, and improvements on PC platforms enable nonvisual play. Major titles incorporate robust audio cues or screen reader pipelines, allowing blind and low-vision (BLV) players to compete alongside sighted peers. Codesign studies and evaluation frameworks tailor feedback to genre conventions, maintaining challenge while improving clarity. However, gaps remain: localization beyond English, prepurchase disclosure of accessibility features, and fair refund policies.

References

1. Frankel, H.L.: Spinal Cord. **50**(11), 790 (2012). https://doi.org/10.1038/sc.2012.109
2. Silver, J.R.: J. Med. Biogr. **20**(3), 101 (2012). https://doi.org/10.1258/jmb.2012.012055
3. Institut Guttmann: History of adapted sport and the institut guttmann. https://www.guttmann.com/en/history-adapted-sport-and-institut-guttmann (2025). Accessed: 2025
4. Schültke, E.: J. Hist. Neurosci. **10**(3), 300 (2001). https://doi.org/10.1076/jhin.10.3.300.9090
5. Britannica: Ludwig guttmann. https://www.britannica.com/biography/Ludwig-Guttmann (2014). Accessed: 2025
6. Paralympic.org: Paralympics history - evolution of the paralympic movement. https://www.paralympic.org/ipc/history (2019). Accessed: 2025
7. Inside the Games: The history of the paralympic movement. https://www.insidethegames.biz/articles/1010776/the-history-of-the-paralympic-movement (2021). Accessed: 2025
8. Paralympic.org: Rome 1960. https://www.paralympic.org/rome-1960 (2019). Accessed: 2025
9. Inside the Games: 1960 - rome. https://www.insidethegames.biz/articles/1010779/1960-rome (2021). Accessed: 2025
10. World Abilitysport: History. https://worldabilitysport.org/about/who-we-are/history/ (2023). Accessed: 2025

11. VIRTUS: Paralympic games. https://virtus.sport/paralympic-games (2025). Accessed: 2025
12. Gold, J.R., Gold, M.M.: J. R. Soc. Promot. Health. **127**(3), 133 (2007)
13. Guttmann, L.: Textbook of Sport for the Disabled. HM&M Publishers. Aylesbury, Bucks, UK. (1976)
14. Paralympic.org: Goalball at the paralympics. https://www.paralympic.org/goalball/about (2025). Accessed: 2025
15. Goulart-Siqueira, G., Benítez-Flores, S., Ferreira, A.R.P., Zagatto, A.M., Foster, C., Boullosa, D.: Heliyon. **6**(7), e04407 (2020). https://doi.org/10.1016/j.heliyon.2020.e04407
16. Molik, B., Morgulec-Adamowicz, N., Kosmol, A., Perkowski, K., Bednarczuk, G., Skowroński, W., Gomez, M.A., Antón, I.C., Szyman, R.J.: J. Hum. Kinet. **48**(1), 43 (2015). https://doi.org/10.1515/hukin-2015-0090
17. Winckler, C., Miranda, A.J.: Aspetar Sports Med. J. **7**, 422 (2018)
18. Nakazawa, K.: Jpn. J. Phys. Fitness Sports Med. **69**(1), 11 (2020)
19. Handi Life Sport: Blind sports. https://handilifesport.com/segments/blind-sports/ (2022). Accessed: 2025
20. Newzoo global games market report 2020. https://newzoo.com/insights/trend-reports/newzoo-global-games-market-report-2020-light-version/
21. Newzoo global games market report 2024. https://newzoo.com/resources/trend-reports/newzoos-global-games-market-report-2024-free-version
22. Tull, M.T., Edmonds, K.A., Scamaldo, K.M., Richmond, J.R., Rose, J.P., Gratz, K.L.: Psychiatry Res. **289**, 113098 (2020)
23. Audiogames.net. https://audiogames.net/
24. Summary wiki: Information on accessible games for the visually impaired. http://mm-galabo.com/AcGameWiki/
25. Yuan, B., Folmer, E., Harris, F.C.: Univ. Access Inf. Soc. **10**, 81 (2011)
26. Porter, J.R., Kientz, J.A.: Proceedings of the 15th International ACM SIGACCESS Conference on Computers and Accessibility, p. 3. ACM, New York, NY, U.S. (2013)
27. de Borba Campos, M., Oliveira, J.D.: International Conference on Universal Access in Human- Computer Interaction, pp. 38–48. Springer, Cham, Switzerland (2016)
28. Westin, T., Ku, J.J., Dupire, J., Hamilton, I.: International Conference on Computers Helping People with Special Needs, pp. 270–279. Springer, Cham, Switzerland (2018)
29. Urbanek, M., Güldenpfennig, F.: Proceedings of the 14th International Audio Mostly Conference: A Journey in Sound, pp. 90–97 (2019)
30. Andrade, R., Rogerson, M.J., Waycott, J., Baker, S., Vetere, F.: Proceedings of the 2019 CHI Conference on Human Factors in Computing Systems, pp. 116:1–14 (2019)
31. Leung, K.M., Chu, W.: PLoS One. **18**(4), e0284504 (2023)
32. Guzmán, D.E., Rengifo, C.F., García-Cena, C.E.: Multimodal Technol. Interact. **8**(8), 64 (2024)
33. Japan eSports Care Association: Manual for using esports in elderly care facilities. https://www.esports-kaigo.org/ (2021)
34. Greenberg Traurig LLP: An overview of the esports market in Japan. https://www.gtlaw.com/en/insights/2022/2/an-overview-of-the-esports-market-in-japan (2022)
35. Smartlaunch: In Japan, esports has become a regular part of treat-ment and rehabilitation regimes. https://smartlaunch.com/in-japan-esports-has-become-a-regular-part-of-treatment-and-rehabilitation-regimes (2024)
36. Mayo Clinic: The Rise of Esports: Caring for Gamers, https://www.mayoclinic.org/mac-20538504 (2022)
37. DiFrancisco-Donoghue, J., Werner, W.G., Douris, P., Zwibel, H.: J. Sport Health Sci. **8**(6), 483 (2019). https://doi.org/10.1016/j.jshs.2019.04.004
38. McNulty, C., Jenny, S.E., Leis, O., Poulus, D., Sondergeld, P., Nicholson, M.: J. Electron. Gaming Esports. **1**(1), 1 (2023). https://doi.org/10.1123/jege.2022-0014
39. DiFrancisco-Donoghue, J., Balentine, J., Schmidt, G., Zwibel, H.: BMJ Open Sport Exerc. Med. **5**(1), e000467 (2019). https://doi.org/10.1136/bmjsem-2018-000467

40. Bavelier, D., Green, C.S.: Curr. Dir. Psychol. Sci. **18**(21), 1881 (2008)
41. Janzen, T.B., Koshimori, Y., Richard, N.M., Thaut, M.H.: Front. Hum. Neurosci. **15**, 789467 (2022). https://doi.org/10.3389/fnhum.2021.789467
42. Bieleke, M., Marczak, M., Engert, V., Mierke, J.: Virtual Real. Exergaming. **29**, 91 (2025). https://doi.org/10.1007/s10055-025-01161-w
43. Miyamoto, T., Kawai, J.: Basics of Coaching Athletes with Visual Impairments (in Japanese). University of Tsukuba Press, Tsukuba, Japan (2021)
44. 2024 ipc classification code (version 29, april 2024). https://www.paralympic.org/sites/default/files/2024-05/IPC_Classification_Code_Version_29_April_2024.pdf
45. Chun, R., Creese, M., Massof, R.W.: Optom. Vis. Sci. **98**(7), 759 (2021)
46. Van Rheden, V., Grah, T., Meschtscherjakov, A.: Proceedings of the 15th International Audio Mostly Conference, pp. 199–205 (2020)
47. Benson, L.C., Räisänen, A.M., Volkova, V.G., Pasanen, K., Emery, C.A.: J. Orthop. Sports Phys. Ther. **50**(10), 549 (2020)
48. Rector, K., Vilardaga, R., Lansky, L., Lu, K., Bennett, C.L., Ladner, R.E., Kientz, J.A.: ACM Trans- actions on Accessible Computing (TACCESS). **9**(4), 1 (2017)
49. Rogge, A.K., Hamacher, D., Cappagli, G., Kuhne, L., Hötting, K., Zech, A., Gori, M., Röder, B.: Exp. Brain Res. **239**(4), 1111 (2021)
50. Zhu, Y., Wang, C., Liu, W., Lv, Y.: Proceedings of the Seventh International Symposium of Chinese CHI, pp. 7–15 (2019)
51. Pieralisi, M., Petrini, V., Di Mattia, V., Manfredi, G., De Leo, A., Scalise, L., Russo, P., Cerri, G.: Sensors. **15**(7), 16466 (2015)
52. Ball, L.E., Lieberman, L.J., Beach, P., Perreault, M., Rich, J.: Int. J. Environ. Res. Public Health. **19**(19), 12907 (2022)
53. Muehlbradt, A., Koushik, V., Kane, S.K.: Proceedings of the 19th International Acm Sigaccess Conference on Computers and Accessibility, pp. 377–378 (2017)
54. Gibelli, E., Morra, D., Gelsomini, M., Matera, M.: Proceedings of the 15th Biannual Conference of the Italian SIGCHI Chapter, pp. 1–8 (2023)
55. Link, D., Weber, C.: PLoS One. **13**(4), e0196679 (2018)
56. Comeras-Chueca, C., Bascuas, P.J., Berzosa, C., Piedrafita, E., Rabal-Pelay, J., Gutiérrez, H., Bataller-Cervero, A.V.: Sports. **12**(11), 291 (2024)
57. Bataller-Cervero, A.V., Bascuas, P.J., Rabal-Pelay, J., Gutiérrez, H., Piedrafita, E., Berzosa, C.: Biology. **11**(8), 1234 (2022)
58. Watanabe, M.: J. Phys. Ther. Sci. **36**(4), 161 (2024)
59. Matsumoto, K., Tanaka, T., Ueda, M.: J. Acoust. Soc. Jpn. **76**(7), 398 (2020)
60. Khurana, R., Wang, A., Carrington, P.: Proceedings of the 23rd International ACM SIGACCESS Conference on Computers and Accessibility, pp. 1–11 (2021)
61. Petrigna, L., Giustino, V., Zangla, D., Aurea, S., Palma, R., Palma, A., Battaglia, G.: Heliyon. **6**, 7 (2020)
62. Karakaya, I.C., Aki, E., Ergun, N.: Percept. Mot. Skills. **108**(1), 129 (2009)
63. Palacín Artigosa, D., Ardigò, L.P., Rico-González, M.: Educ. Sci. **12**(10), 714 (2022)
64. Makaracı, Y., Nas, K., Pamuk, Ö., Aydemir, M.: J. Exerc. Rehabil. **18**(5), 308 (2022)
65. Alves, I.d.S., Kalva-Filho, C.A., Aquino, R., Travitzki, L., Tosim, A., Papoti, M., Morato, M. P.: Front. Physiol. **9**, 1636 (2018)
66. Gökşen, A., Ince, G., Alcan, V.: BMC Sports Sci. Med. Rehabil. **16**(1), 99 (2024)
67. Larsen, C.H.: J. Sport Psychol. Action. **5**(3), 186 (2014)
68. Miura, T., Soga, S., Matsuo, M., Sakajiri, M., Onishi, J., Ono, T.: Proceedings of the 9th Augmented Human International Conference, pp. 1–5 (2018)
69. Watanabe, M., Miura, T., Matsuo, M., Sakajiri, M., Onishi, J.: Computers Helping People with Special Needs: 18th International Conference, ICCHP-AAATE 2022, Lecco, Italy, July 11–15, 2022, Proceedings, Part II, pp. 79–88. Springer, Cham, Switzerland (2022)
70. Blauert, J.: Spatial Hearing: The Psychophysics of Human Sound Localization. MIT Press (1997)

71. Cairns, P., Power, C., Barlet, M., Haynes, G., Kaufman, C., Beeston, J.: Games Cult. **16**(2), 262 (2021)
72. Agrimi, E., Battaglini, C., Bottari, D., Gnecco, G., Leporini, B.: Soft. Comput. **28**(17), 10475 (2024)
73. Strobel, L., Gerling, K.: ACM Trans. Comput.-Hum. Interact. (2025)
74. Yuan, B., Folmer, E.: Proceedings of the 10th International ACM SIGACCESS Conference on Computers and Accessibility, pp. 169–176 (2008)
75. Gaudy, T., Natkin, S., D.: Archambault. In: Transactions on Edutainment II, pp. 176–186. Springer, Cham, Switzerland (2009)
76. Sánchez, J., Sáenz, M., Pascual-Leone, A., Merabet, L.: CHI'10 Extended Abstracts on Human Factors in Computing Systems, pp. 3409–3414 (2010)
77. Sánchez, J., Sáenz, M., Pascual-Leone, A., Merabet, L.: CHI'10 Extended Abstracts on Human Factors in Computing Systems, pp. 3991–3996 (2010)
78. L.B. Merabet, E.C. Connors, M.A. Halko, J. Sánchez, (2012)
79. Connors, E.C., Yazzolino, L.A., Sánchez, J., Merabet, L.B.: J. Vis. Exp. (73), 50272 (2013)
80. Connors, E.C., Chrastil, E.R., Sánchez, J., Merabet, L.B.: Front. Hum. Neurosci. **8**, 133 (2014)
81. Garcia, F.E., de Almeida Neris, V.P.: International Conference on Human-Computer Interaction, pp. 229–238. Springer, Cham, Switzerland (2013)
82. Balan, O., Moldoveanu, A., Moldoveanu, F.: Int. J. Disabil. Hum. Dev. **14**(2), 109 (2015)
83. Chavez Sanchez, F., de La Peña, G.A.M., Adriana Mendoza Franco, G., Iroel Heredia Carrillo, E.: Proceedings of the 16th International Audio Mostly Conference, pp. 24–31 (2021)
84. Mrazik, M., Khatib, F.: ACM Games Res. Pract. **2**(4), 1 (2024)
85. Morelli, T., Foley, J., Columna, L., Lieberman, L., Folmer, E.: Proceedings of the Fifth International Conference on the Foundations of Digital Games, pp. 147–154 (2010)
86. Morelli, T., Foley, J., Folmer, E.: Proceedings of the 12th International ACM SIGACCESS Conference on Computers and Accessibility, pp. 179–186 (2010)
87. Morelli, T., Foley, J., Lieberman, L., Folmer, E.: Proceedings of Graphics Interface 2011, pp. 223–230 (2011)
88. Morelli, T., Lieberman, L., Foley, J., Folmer, E.: FDG (2014)
89. Morelli, T., Folmer, E.: Entertain. Comput. **5**(1), 83 (2014)
90. Nair, V., Karp, J.L., Silverman, S., Kalra, M., Lehv, H., Jamil, F., Smith, B.A.: The 34th Annual ACM Symposium on User Interface Software and Technology, pp. 538–551 (2021)
91. Gonçalves, D., Piĉarra, M., Pais, P., Guerreiro, J., Rodrigues, A.: Proceedings of the 2023 CHI Conference on Human Factors in Computing Systems, pp. 1–15 (2023)
92. Leite, P.d.S., Almeida, L.D.A.: International Conference on Human-Computer Interaction, pp. 166–185. Springer (2021)
93. Larreina-Morales, M.E.: Games Cult. **19**(1), 75 (2024)
94. Matsuo, M., Miura, T., Yabu, K., Katagiri, A., Sakajiri, M., Onishi, J., Kurata, T., Ifukube, T.: Proceedings of the 2021 International Conference on Multimodal Interaction, pp. 62–70 (2021)
95. Miura, T., Matsuo, M., Yabu, K., Katagiri, A., Sakajiri, M., Onishi, J., Kurata, T., Ifukube, T.: Proceedings of the ACM on Interactive, Mobile, Wearable and Ubiquitous Technologies. **4**(4), 1 (2020)
96. Gnecco, G., Battaglini, C., Biancalani, F., Bottari, D., Camurri, A., Leporini, B.: International Conference on Intelligent Technologies for Interactive Entertainment, pp. 167–177. Springer, Cham, Switzerland (2023)
97. Matsuo, M., Miura, T., Sakajiri, M., Onishi, J., Ono, T.: International Conference on Computers Helping People with Special Needs, pp. 537–544. Springer, Cham, Switzerland (2016)
98. Matsuo, M., Sakajiri, M., Onishi, J., Ono, T., Miura, T.: J. Technol. Pers. Disabil. **5**, 172 (2017)
99. Potluri, V., Vaithilingam, P., Iyengar, S., Vidya, Y., Swaminathan, M., Srinivasa, G.: Proceedings of the 2018 Chi Conference on Human Factors in Computing Systems, pp. 1–11 (2018)

100. Baker, C.M., Milne, L.R., Ladner, R.E.: Proceedings of the 33rd Annual ACM Conference on Human Factors in Computing Systems, pp. 3043–3052 (2015)
101. Ehtesham-Ul-Haque, M., Monsur, S.M., Billah, S.M.: Proceedings of the 35th Annual ACM Symposium on User Interface Software and Technology, pp. 1–21 (2022)
102. Miura, T., Fujii, H., Yamazaki, R., Erdenesambuu, D., Matsuo, M., Sakajiri, M., Onishi, J.: J. Technol. Pers. Disabil, 184–196 (2024)
103. Stadler, V., Hlavacs, H.: Proceedings of the 2018 Annual Symposium on Computer-Human Interaction in Play, pp. 503–509 (2018)
104. Martinez, J.J., Froehlich, J.E., Fogarty, J.: Proceedings of the 2024 CHI Conference on Human Factors in Computing Systems, pp. 1–17 (2024)
105. Hammad, N., Elavsky, F., Moharana, S., Chen, J., Lee, S., Carrington, P., Moritz, D., Hammer, J., Harpstead, E.: Proceedings of the 26th International ACM SIGACCESS Conference on Computers and Accessibility, pp. 1–13 (2024)
106. Ran, Z., Li, X., Xiao, Q., Fan, X., Li, F.M., Wang, Y., Lu, Z.: Proceedings of the 2025 CHI Conference on Human Factors in Computing Systems, pp. 1–18 (2025)
107. Sodhi, P., Girouard, A., Thue, D.: Companion Proceedings of the Annual Symposium on Computer-Human Interaction in Play, pp. 49–55 (2023)
108. Matsuo, M., Erdenesambuu, D., Sakajiri, M., Onishi, J., Miura, T.: International Conference on Computers Helping People with Special Needs, pp. 128–136. Springer, Cham, Switzerland (2024)
109. Matsuo, M., Kitamura, N., Egashira, M., Hosogai, T., Hatakeyama, S., Kato, D., Hayakawa, K., Onishi, J., Sakajiri, M., Miura, T.: International Conference on Computers Helping People with Special Needs, pp. 137–145. Springer, Cham, Switzerland (2024)

MIX
Papier aus verantwortungsvollen Quellen
Paper from responsible sources
FSC® C105338

If you have any concerns about our products,
you can contact us on
ProductSafety@springernature.com

In case Publisher is established outside the EU,
the EU authorized representative is:
Springer Nature Customer Service Center GmbH
Europaplatz 3, 69115 Heidelberg, Germany

Printed by Libri Plureos GmbH
in Hamburg, Germany